SpringerBriefs in Molecular Science

Chemistry of Foods

Series editor

Salvatore Parisi, Palermo, Italy

More information about this series at http://www.springer.com/series/11853

Giovanni Brunazzi · Salvatore Parisi
Amina Pereno

The Importance of Packaging Design for the Chemistry of Food Products

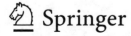 Springer

Giovanni Brunazzi
Brunazzi & Associati
Turin
Italy

Amina Pereno
Department of Architecture and Design
Politecnico di Torino
Turin
Italy

Salvatore Parisi
Industrial Consultant
Palermo
Italy

ISSN 2191-5407　　　　　ISSN 2191-5415　(electronic)
ISBN 978-3-319-08451-0　ISBN 978-3-319-08452-7　(eBook)
DOI 10.1007/978-3-319-08452-7

Library of Congress Control Number: 2014942663

Springer Cham Heidelberg New York Dordrecht London

Printed on acid-free paper

Springer is part of Springer Science+Business Media (www.springer.com)

Contents

Chapter 1
Introduction

Abstract Visible features of packaged foods are mainly influenced by packaging: the necessity of separating the exterior 'wrap' from the contained object should be highlighted. In fact, packaging is often perceived such as the carrier of subliminal messages with peculiar and designable meanings and suggestions. As a result, packaged foods may be differently perceived by normal users depending on the physical appearance of packaging. Most common food pack have always been designed and produced with several specific aims: the easy classification of foods from the marketing viewpoint; the reliable subdivision of apparently similar food products in sub-classes; the constant reference to implicit properties and safety features. Moreover, the problem of storage conditions and the possibility of using FP as 'cooking' or 'serving' devices can undoubtedly make more difficult the packaging design. Therefore, food packaging should be well examined by chemical and design viewpoints. Chemistry influences designers, and design models also the chemical nature of FP. This loop mechanism can modify the final packaged food with notable implications.

Keywords Food packaging · Integrated food product · Communication design · Normal consumer · Packaging design · Food brand

Abbreviations

FP   Food packaging
IFP   Integrated food product

© The Author(s) 2014   1
G. Brunazzi et al., *The Importance of Packaging Design for the Chemistry of Food Products*, SpringerBriefs in Chemistry of Foods,
DOI: 10.1007/978-3-319-08452-7_1

1.1 Appearance and Substance: Several Preliminary Observations on Packaging

At present, the redundant presence of stereotypes sometimes darkens the complexity of the real world: things, situations and concepts.

In fact, the well known motto '*Appearances are deceptive*' and similar observations highlight the necessity of separating the exterior 'wrap' from the contained object. Normally, this assumption is considered reliable when speaking of daily and ordinary objects in the modern world: the 'wrap' is often perceived as a carrier of subliminal messages with mendacious or reliable meanings and suggestions. Anyway, this meaningful function can be designable and modifiable. The simple suspect of this possibility may be very disturbing for normal people.

From the anthropological point of view, every human culture has always expressed the desire of 'dressing' living bodies and, often, material things. At the same time, it should be evident that all types of sumptuous or shabby 'covering' device mean and denote a multiplicity of functional exigencies and intangible concepts at the same time. In other words, packaging may express simple 'covering roles' and more profound, but unexpressed, functions: relationships between different human cultures, symbolic messages to the individual and collective unconscious of the local communities.

Other important considerations can be elaborated from the sociological viewpoint. The basic aim of this book is related to foods and the chemistry of these products, focusing on their packaging design. The necessity of preserving liquid and solid foods is ancient. After all, great religions have always underlined, with minute and intensely prescriptive care, both the nutritional and the sacred values of foods. Symbolic meanings and social identity references are surely represented in every food product. The careful observance of Jewish diet prescriptions and other traditional texts can demonstrate the importance of the attribution of non-edible properties to food products and related diets. Every simple prescription can appear functional for a 'technical' description of foods and their own origin, even if the shown justification is purely religious and related to the 'purity' of the observant person.

Nowadays, gastronomic traditions may clearly identify the regional identity, similarly to the languages and related behaviours. This approach appears the last tenacious barrier against the development of the 'universal globalisation' of the modern economy.

Certainly, a number of 'poor' food products (expression of regional areas with peculiar connotations such as economic instability, recurrent famines and reduced variability of basic ingredients) have been progressively modified without peculiar packaging features. However, this assumption does not appear necessarily truthful.

Indeed, some of most known food packaging (FP) in the western world of 50 or 60 years ago showed interesting peculiarities with concern to external properties, their appearance and correlated 'technological' functions. It should be difficult to propose faithfully the same type of FP in the present world, certainly more opulent and un-weakened by the risk of famines and durable wars. Common sugar commodities were packaged in simple (but extremely functional) blue paper; on the other hand, meat products were presented in yellow paper only. This simple colorimetric denotation, apparently subordinate to aesthetical preferences or gastronomic properties of contained foods, had instead the implicit aim of defining a sort of general, reliable and 'universal' chromatic code without apparent misunderstandings. Most common packages for the harvesting of animal milk, bottles for vegetable oils and for wines were 'designed' and produced with the same intention: to offer the best answer to following functional needs:

- The reliable classification of foods, from the marketing viewpoint.
- The subdivision of apparently similar food products in sub-classes.
- The constant and reliable reference to the chemical composition and the microbial ecology, often and gladly only implicit, of foods.
- The necessity of using proper FP for food preservation, with a preliminary choice between those available materials (paper, metals, glass).

FP have to comply today with a series of hygiene and safety standards in addition to the implicit and basic prerequisite: the mere preservation of foods. Moreover, the problem of storage conditions and the possibility of using FP as 'cooking' or 'serving' devices can undoubtedly complicate the packaging design [1, 2].

Finally, it has to be necessarily recognised that FP is a fundamental vector for the commercial identification and the success of food products for extended time periods: in other words, the strategy of 'visual communication' must be elaborated with the choice of the 'best' FP [3, 4]. Naturally, every vector should be linked to a peculiar food and one single brand only, with well recognisable features, despite unpredictable failures can occur [5–7].

It has been reported that food and non food products were produced and sold without precise marketing descriptions in several Countries such as the old Soviet Union, because of the concept of collective and planned economy: in other words, competition between different articles was really difficult because official prices were mainly set for satisfying distributional objectives instead of ration supply [8]. On these bases, it could be inferred that the most evident function of food- and non-food packaging is linked to the communication of packaged products [9, 10].

However, our impressions may be simpler than the reality. In fact, the research of a personal (induced or planned) feature can still demonstrate the individuality of single persons, designers and users, despite tacit objections: anyway, the decisional autonomy would be already serially programmed.

On the other side, more pressing reasons can influence the nature of the packaged food or beverage, also definable as the 'integrated food product' (IFP) [3]. This definition means the sum of the packaged (preserved) food and other accessory, visible or invisible, features.

In fact, the whole design process of packaged foods and beverages starts from three main basic concepts: the final use (of the product), the final user (the consumer) and the final price. This approach leads to design and diversify similar products in order to meet the requirements of different users. Different products mean different packaging, with specific features from the chemical and technological viewpoint: every food is technology, history, tradition, culture, regulatory … and chemistry also.

For example, with concern to different subtypes of the same original product within a single food plant, the simple variation of one or two points in the initial formula or ingredient list can surely determine important and desirable modifications in the final result. Actually, main and secondary analytical features of examined products—water, fat matter, carbohydrates, oxidisable vitamins, colorimetrically active compounds, microelements, etc.—may be subjected to important variations because of the mutation of original formulations and/or unavoidable chemical reactions during the 'shelf life' period. Different causes or synergic reasons may mean different results; consequently, similar but unalike IFP should be expected.

Above mentioned reflections concern several thematic areas of the whole world of food technology, including FP also. It has to be noted that the initial and aware (or 'induced') choice of the final user has to be confirmed and 'reassured' before and after the purchase. The first appearance of IFP is mainly influenced by FP: printed images and logos, the perception of brightness or the total transparency of wraps, basic tactile sensations… and other factors should be considered also. These features can be obtained thanks to the different chemical properties of FP and the succession of various production processes. All FP features can surely influence the choice of users—final targets of the whole process—in a positive way.

On the other side, the use of a peculiar FP can also be linked to IFP food failures [3]. Actually, these defects can be directly or indirectly connected to FP: the common point appears at least related to chemistry. In fact, packaged foods are partially or totally 'hidden' by means of FP: as a result, basic organoleptic perceptions of IFP can be slightly altered, but the alteration should be considered in both directions.

For example, final consumers may be aware that their preferred IFP is not always 'constant' because of normal variations in the compositional list of ingredients. The variability of seasons, predictable or sudden scarcity periods and other economic factors may alter basic perceptions (tastes, odours, texture, colours, general aspect) of purchased packaged foods. However, the same reasoning concerns FP also: recurrent economic depressions can suddenly increase prices of raw materials, including plastic matters, metals, etc., with natural variations in the chemical composition of FP. However, consumers seem oddly unaware of this important aspect.

As a consequence, it should be concluded FP is the main media to show the food product: this important and basic factor of the synergic IFP should be well examined by chemical and packaging design viewpoints at the same time. Chemistry influences designers, and Design models the chemical nature of FP; according to the motto '*Better Design for a Better Food*', this loop mechanism can modify the final IFP with notable implications.

Obviously, the choice of a single portioned product is not a sort of declaration of independence of the final consumer. On the other side, it should be noted that the personal freedom of people can be found and hidden beyond the little dimension of FP, the soft occasion of the purchase, the consequent repetition of the same act. This choice and the original determination or consumeristic freedom is surely modifiable and metastable: the same thing can be affirmed with relation to the market of food products. As a clear consequence, all IFP elements—including FP also—should be studied to discover invisible connections between this 'principle of self-determination' of consumers and the designed capability of IFP to become adherent to different behavioural types. The basic aim of this book is to conjugate this peculiar approach with industrial possibilities of the current world of IFP from a typical chemical viewpoint.

References

1. Piergiovanni L, Limbo S (2010) Materiali, tecnologie e qualità degli alimenti. Springer-Verlag Italia, Milan
2. Marsh K, Bugusu B (2007) Food packaging—roles, materials, and environmental issues. J Food Sci 72(3):39–55. doi:10.1111/j.1750-3841.2007.00301.x
3. Parisi S (2012) Food packaging and food alterations: the user-oriented approach. Smithers Rapra Technology, Shawbury
4. De Nardo LM (2009) Food packaging: designing with the consumer. Elledì, Milan
5. Parisi S (2004) Alterazioni in imballaggi metallici termicamente processati. Gulotta Press, Palermo
6. Brunazzi G (2009) Hello! Logos. Logos, Modena
7. Margolin V (2013) Design studies and food studies: parallels and intersections. Des Cult 5(3):375–392. doi:10.2752/175470813X13705953612327
8. Tyers R (1994) Economic reform in Europe and the former Soviet Union: implications for international food markets. Research report 99, Intl Food Policy Res Inst (IFPRI), Research report 99, Washington, DC, p 12
9. Parisi S (2005) New implications of packaging in food products. Food Package Bull 14(8 & 9): 2–5
10. Volli U (2012) Semiotica della pubblicità. Laterza, Rome

Chapter 2
Packaging and Food: A Complex Combination

Abstract The advent of packaging materials in the modern food industry has deeply changed the relationship between people and foods. Food packages have progressively been turned into essential element for the sale and the consumption of food products. On these bases, packaged foods can become communicative media of values and information: the user receives and understands these data by means of suitable tools of physical, cultural and personal nature. Functional and communicative requirements of food packaging are continuously evolving: the careful analysis of these factors should be recommended because of their influence on chemistry of foods, food technology, biochemical interactions between different food phases, and chemistry of food packaging. This section is dedicated to the study and the 'chemical' interpretation of food packaging requirements.

Keywords Food packaging · Communication · Regulatory · Food consumption · Packaging design · Recycling

Abbreviations

BOPP	Biaxially oriented polypropylene
BRC	British retail consortium
Cr_2O_3	Chromium oxide
DOS	Dioctyl sebacate
ECCS	Electrolytic chromium oxide coated steel
ETP	Electrolytic tin plate
EVA	Ethylene vinyl acetate
EVOH	Ethylene vinyl alcohol
EFSA	European food safety authority
EU	European Union
EPS	Expanded polystyrene
FU	Final user
FIFO	First in first out
FP	Food packaging
FM	Food manufacturer
FPM	Food packaging material

© The Author(s) 2014

G. Brunazzi et al., *The Importance of Packaging Design for the Chemistry of Food Products*, SpringerBriefs in Chemistry of Foods,
DOI: 10.1007/978-3-319-08452-7_2

FPP	Food packaging producer
FSSC	Food safety system certification
GSFS	Global standard for food safety
BRC/IOP	Global standard for packaging and packaging materials
GMP	Good manufacturing practice
HACCP	Hazard analysis and critical control points
H_2S	Hydrogen sulphide
HDPE	High density polyethylene
HIPS	High impact polystyrene
IoP	Institute of Packaging
IFP	Integrated food product
IFS	International Featured Standard
ISO	International Organisation for Standardisation
IUPAC	International Union of Pure and Applied Chemistry
Fe_2O_3	Iron oxide
ITX	Isopropyl thioxanthone
JIT	Just in time
LIFO	Last in first out
LLDPE	Linear low-density polyethylene
LDPE	Low density polyethylene
MAP	Modified atmosphere packaging
MW	Molecular weight
NIAS	Non-intentionally added substance
OBA	Optical brightness agents
OPP	Oriented polypropylene
P&B	Paper and Board
PA	Polyamides
PE	Polyethylene
PET, PETE	Polyethylene terephthalate
PP	Polypropylene
PS	Polystyrene
PVC	Polyvinyl chloride
PVDC	Polyvinylidene chloride
RFID	Radio frequency identification
REACH	Registration, evaluation, authorisation and restriction of chemicals
SBB	Solid bleached board
SBB	Solid unbleached board
TFS	Tin free steel
UV	Ultraviolet
ZnO	Zinc oxide

2.1 Packaging and Food: An Introduction

The historical evolution of commercial products is strictly connected with the concomitant evolution of packaging: container tools and contained goods are components of the same inseparable unit. This link is surely stronger and meaningful in the field of foods and beverages because of the notable symbolic value of food products [1].

The advent of packaging in the modern food industry has caused fundamental transformations with concern to the relationship between people and foods. As a result, food packaging (FP) has progressively been turned into an essential element for the sale and the consumption of the food product [2]. In fact, foods are not exclusively perceived as primary needs by final consumers. The simple eating act is now the expression of strong cultural and ethical values in the current economic context without the risk of sudden famines. Actually, the main problem of the modern world is the overproduction of industrial commodities in several economic cycles and areas.

As a consequence, foods are not different from other consumer goods: this concept is obligatorily correlated to the consumption activity and communication features. Substantially, consumption is not always a mere purchasing activity. Final users (FU) are often used or 'forced' to externalise their personality on purchased goods, even if the unconscious projection of one's own attitudes and feelings is not complete. On these bases, every good or service can become a communication media of values and information: the user receives and understands these data by means of suitable tools of physical, cultural and personal nature [3].

Foods and beverages are often perceived as vehicles of contradictory values and behaviours:

- The hedonistic idea of the maximum pleasure of tastes and the obsessive negation of unpleasant effects on the human being
- The rapidity of individual meals and the pleasure of the conviviality
- The necessity of ready-to-eat products and the increasing attention to healthy foods.

In addition, many urgent topics affect both the regulatory and the social viewpoints: hygiene and safety discussions are essential matters.

FP is the first communicative element of the 'integrated food product' (IFP). The final user is used to expect, see and recognise the exteriority of IPF before other important and meaningful elements, including the real edible content. This mechanism is the most probable behaviour in the modern context of the mass retailing industry: self-service seems the general rule [4]. On these bases, FP should answer to expressed and implicit questions, doubts and needs of FU. As a consequence, FP may become the real intermediary between the food manufacturer (FM), the mass retailer and the FU. Moreover, FP has to comply with peculiar functional features with concern to usability, storage and transportation [5–7].

It is known that functional factors and the communication features are the most important requirements for FP: however, the complex process of packaging design cannot be easily and roughly circumscribed to these aspects. Regulatory requirements concerning FP and food packaging materials (FPM) are more and more urgent and specific: technological roles are constantly examined and reviewed, but other obligations have been recently introduced or suggested. Nutritional labelling measures in the European Union (EU) are certainly good examples. Additionally, packaging designers have to comply with other needs such as the increasing attention to the environmental policy and the sustainable management of resources and wastes.

However, the above-mentioned topics cannot be discussed without the fundamental role of chemistry and technology: the advent of plastic matters in the industry of packaging has completely and irreversibly transformed the concept of FP with unpredictable results [2, 8].

An important aspect is correlated to the geographical availability of certain materials, chemical intermediates and suitable structures for the production of FP. On the other side, packaging can be simply assembled in a few favoured locations fitting together parts, intermediates and chemicals from different geographical areas. This is the natural consequence of the effective (or excessive) industrial specialization in several countries.

The above-mentioned situation should be carefully considered when speaking of food failures and possible contamination events. Several of most recent food scandals may be investigated by this viewpoint [9]: in fact, certain chemical analytes may be (a) absent in food production sites and (b) present near FP plants at the same time. Moreover, the conceptual displacement of FP components can complicate the investigation: every packaging may be seen as a single container with 'n' parts or chemical intermediates/raw materials from 'n' different locations. As a result, every food contamination by FP could have been originated only by one of 'n' different sites.

This consideration should be taken into account when considering chemical contamination and microbiological dangers also. For example, the occurrence of microbial outbreaks with heavy consequences for human safety has been recently correlated with the environmental contamination of packaging machinery into food companies [10]. Once more, the role of FP can be considered of basic importance when speaking of food preservation and food failures.

Anyway, functional and communicative requisites of FP are continuously evolving: the careful analysis of these factors should be recommended because of their influence on the structure and the behaviour of the future IFP. This investigation is mainly based on chemical-physical features of IFP: chemistry of foods, food technology, biochemical interactions between different food phases ... and chemistry of food packaging [10]. In fact, chemistry of FP can influence heavily the future IFP.

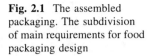

Fig. 2.1 The assembled packaging. The subdivision of main requirements for food packaging design

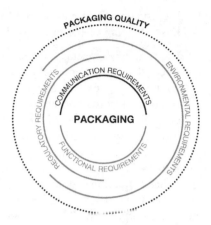

However, the above-mentioned analysis should highlight and clarify existing connections between the chemical features of IPF and complex of PF requirements. This study may appear complicated because of the apparent dissimilarity between two worlds: the materialistic and 'scientifically exact' physicality of chemistry on the one hand, and the creativity of design science on the other side. Apparently, two different and irreconcilable visions of the world are shown here.

First of all, the whole group of food packaging design requirements should be divided into four macro categories, as shown in Fig. 2.1:

1. Functional requirements
2. Communicative requirements
3. Regulatory requirements
4. Environmental requirements

However, similar categories are strictly correlated with important juxtapositions during the whole life of the final IPF and FP.

The complete compliance of all requirements is fundamental with relation to the quality of the final FP and the efficacy of design. Different requirements have different importance depending on the final IFP and correlated production processes. Because of the main objective of this book, every requirement with potential influence on foods and related physicochemical features will be discussed and connected with the correspondent design action because of the strict relationship between chemistry and functional performances of IPF and FP.

2.2 Functional Requirements

At present, FP has to comply with different and increasing functional needs: the so-called 'globalisation' of markets and the consequent broadening of the whole 'market arena' have transformed the original packaging into a multifunctional instrument with different responsibilities [11]:

- Preservation of contained foods when assembled to obtain the IFP, and
- Easy shipping of the produced IFP in different and remote markets.

The situation appears complex and FP plays one of the most important roles in the food chain [5]. Perishable foods—fruits, vegetables, and so on—have to be preserved during extended time periods and on long distances. Moreover, the continuous and possibly laborious delivery of food commodities (raw materials, intermediates and final IFP) may be fractionated and carried out by different operators. Frozen products have to be obligatorily stored under—18 °C, while refrigerated IFP should remain constantly stored in accordance to less rigorous conditions (the so-called 'cold chain': $2° \pm 2$ °C in several countries). On the other hand, fractionated storage may be carried out with sudden changes in temperature (thermal leaps) and FP have to minimise chemical and microbiological alterations where possible and predictable (mechanical damages should be considered also).

The request and the diffusion of ready-to-eat and pre-cooked foods have also forced packaging producers to create packaging with new features. These FP should be easily opened, possibly usable for sectioning foods and highly resistant to high temperatures when placed into conventional or microwave ovens. With relation to the third feature, FP should not alter contained foods: as a result, every possible chemical reaction at the food/packaging interface should be predicted and possibly avoided. The same thing has to be affirmed when speaking of potential chemical migration of certain analytes, plastic components or possible decomposed matters from FP to foods. Actually, the opposite situation may occur with 'grotesque' results and possible alarming reactions by normal consumers [10].

Another notable question remains to be discussed when considering predictable or unexpected reactions between FP and foods, with reference to predicted performances: the problem of shelf life values. In other words, every packaged food has its own labelled features, including the related durability: this term means the so-called expiration date or 'date of minimum durability' as intended in the EU according to the Council Directive No 2000/13/EC on labelling, presentation and advertising of foodstuffs.

IFP are subject to food degradation because of predictable or unexpected chemical, physical and microbiological degradations, according to the principle of food degradation [5]. Consequently, FP have to preserve packaged foods without the decrease of predictable or calculated shelf life values.

Finally, it should be remembered that different customers can purchase IFP: normal consumers are surely the most important and recognisable target for FM. On the other hand, the 'food and feed chain' is composed of different players, also called 'stakeholders', and some of these subjects is contemporarily producer (of raw materials, intermediated foods or final IFP) and 'user' (of raw materials, or intermediated foods). With exclusive concern to these professional users, the list of requirements for purchased IFP and for every sub-component, including FP, can slightly differ from basic needs of the user. Following requests have to be considered:

- Effective storage systems
- Easier management of the peculiar IFP on shelves near mass retailers
- Increased availability of new and intuitive logistic systems, from the 'First In, First Out' (FIFO) strategy to most recent 'Last In, First Out' (LIFO) and 'Just in Time' (JIT) approaches.

All the earlier discussed points can help to define the whole group of FP requirements: in fact, these factors can be determined by both the main features of the food product (to protect- to transport- to preserve- to store) and the peculiar target (normal consumer, stakeholder and public authorities for food safety).

2.2.1 Preservation and Protection Requirements

Food preservation and food protection are similar concepts. Actually, the first of these definitions is related to the defence of the food product from internal agents and external factors that could enhance food degradation (microbial spreading and degrading chemical reactions such as oxidation or enzymatic browning). Instead, food protection is related to the possible preservation of the whole IFP in every location and during extended temporal periods. Normally, protection requirements concern essentially the defence of the IFP against:

- External physical agents: ultraviolet (UV) rays; powders; compression; crashes; thermal leaps; and
- External chemical agents: environmental moisture; toxic or harmful substances; other chemical contaminants; etc.

One or all of these causes can attack and damage IFP with hygienic problems and/or simple degrading failures: the first and most exposed barrier is naturally the used FP.

On these bases, the initial design of FP and subsequent developments play always a fundamental role with reference to the preservation and the protection of IFP. FP must 'transfer' their peculiar features to the packaged product. Mechanical resistance, flexibility, rigidity, impermeability, gaseous diffusion and less known properties (superficial roughness, porosity, etc.) are surely welcome and desired when the final IFP has to be 'combined' with a sort of chemical and physical impenetrability [12, 13]. Moreover, shapes and sizes are fundamental if packaged products have to be adequately preserved and protected at least from the date of packaging to the end of the minimum durability. Substantially, chemical and technological properties of materials can be enhanced with the 'right' and 'sustainable' choice of the most adaptable shape and/or volumetric capacity [2, 14]. For example, the simple preservation of certain packaged products (FPM: paper and board) against sudden impacts may be notably ameliorated with the correct placement of the food into adequate shapes [15]. It can be assumed that the chemistry of materials is of basic importance for the future performance of FP. The known correlation between the stability of paper and board boxes and certain chemical properties of original FP components (example: dimension, thickness, strength, adhesive power and chemical nature of glues) is a useful example. On the other hand, the chemical nature or FP has to be adaptable to physicochemical features of foods.

Finally, modern closure and opening systems are important elements for the durable protection (impermeability) of IFP against physicochemical agents. In contrast, preservation requirements are mainly related to the protection against microbiological agents: degrading micro organisms (yeasts, moulds, etc.) and pathogenic bacteria [15, 16]. Once more, FP components and original raw materials can play an important role because of the theoretical asepsis of the final container. The same concept has to be repeated when closure systems are created, developed, studied and introduced with the aim of transforming the original food—with its own microbial ecology—into an aseptic, impermeable and 'inviolable' structure.

Actually, the modern FP does not seem to be designed with protective features only: new materials have been recently introduced and developed with innovative features. The most important of these 'enhancements' appears related to the active behaviour of new systems, at present. For example, the so-called 'active packaging' systems are intentionally designed with the aim of enhancing the durability of packaged foods by means of chemical interactions at the food/packaging interface [17, 18].

As a result, it appears that preservation and protection may be obtained at the same time by means of different strategies when speaking of modern packaged foods. However, a useful reflection should be made about unpredictable results of design strategies.

UV rays are known to be active catalysers of microbial spreading and physicochemical reactions (causes: augment of inner temperatures into certain FP; enzymatic reactions; etc.). As a consequence, the above-mentioned design strategies—materials, volumetric capacity, closure systems, and shapes—have to be studied and adapted to every peculiar situation. With reference to this approach, an additional risk is linked to the possible and avoidable damage of the resulting FP by means of packaging strategies. In other words, every design activity is 'forced' to express one or more clear lines of action, while other more or less promising strategies could be judged negatively and preventively eliminated.

Should the 'right' approach be applied to more than one specific situation, normal consumers and official authorities could be obliged to observe predictable failures and consequent hygiene and safety concerns [10, 19, 20]. It may be assumed that every food needs its own active or passive FP [21]: this time, the problem can be originated by the incorrect design and/or incorrect information by FM [5].

2.2.2 *Requirements for Transportation and Storage*

The most part of packaged foods are the last step of a long 'food chain'. In spite of the increasing sensibility towards ethical and environmental topics and the attention for new concepts—short food chain, aware of consumption in favour of local productions and 'low footprint' impact—the food chain is located everywhere on a macroscopic and worldwide scale. As a logical consequence, this situation implies the careful design of IFP and related components, including FP. In other terms, design should take into account the possibility of long distance-transports and possible intermediate storages near 'temporary' loading platforms between the starting point—FM—and the final destination—mass retailers, other marketplaces, and fairs [22].

Every packaging is (a) stored near the food packaging producer (FPP), (b) delivered to the final user (FU) and finally (c) stored by FM (with peculiar and probably different procedures if compared to FPP's advices).

Subsequently, the subject of storage and transportation steps is not FP, but the final IFP: this item is (d) stored near the food industry, (e) delivered to the final destination and finally (f) stored until the use or the purchase by common users [5, 14]. It should be highlighted that:

- The subject of the above-mentioned steps is completely changed
- The delivery step may be often subdivided in two or more intermediate sub-steps between steps (f) and (g) with annexed 'intermediate' or 'temporary' storages near different warehouses.

Consequently, the whole chain of transportation can become complex and probably 'long': every step or sub-step can surely increase the probability of damages (mechanical ruptures, microbial spreading, chemical reactions by heat or UV rays-exposure etc.). In addition, the diversification between different warehouses should be highlighted because of dissimilar storage protocols, distinct managers and so on. From the theoretical viewpoint, it may be assumed that a generic food commodity is subdivided in 'n' different storage warehouses at the final stage just before the purchase. In these conditions, the risk of 'n' or less different behaviours of the same IFP can be predicted with relation to the remaining shelf life (RSL) and correlated original features (colour, aroma, aspect, texture and taste). At present, this discussion is extremely important and 'thorny' [10]. After all, the significance of sampled products for statistical analyses and official examinations may be potentially lowered.

As a result, different exigencies can be discussed when speaking of food transportation and storage; these needs are also correlated to several players of the food chain and different warehousing systems [23]. Anyway, the most influential factors appear to be (a) weight, (b) shape and (c) volumetric capacity: naturally, these features are mainly established in the design step for FP and IFP.

With reference to the primary FP, main challenges appear:

- The definition of the lowest volumetric capacity
- The research of adaptable materials, with some preference for flexible plastics and composite packaging
- The design of protection systems with low encumbrance. Examples: strengthening of lateral ribs; air injection (because of shockproof and insulating properties).

With concern to the secondary packaging, it has to be considered that this container depends strictly on the number and shape of theoretically equal IFP. In fact, every secondary packaging gathers 'n' individual IFP. There is the general opinion that secondary packaging could be more adaptable to different IFP. As a consequence, cardboard (or plastic) boxes are often produced with several standardised sizes only and widely used. On the one hand, the normal placement on single and standardised wooden pallets is surely easier. On the other, available spaces may be irrationally occupied into warehouses, and standardised boxes may be not easily storable onto metallic shelves.

The lack of spaces all around secondary packages can be negatively considered when the so-called 'Hazard Analysis and Critical Control Points' (HACCP) approach is required. In fact, the exposure of IFP to heat, UV rays and other external agents with some degrading importance may be increased if food products are not properly stored: a minimum space around cardboard and plastic boxes should be needed. According to several operators, every 'surrounded' cardboard box should require 20 to 30 cm of free space. This empirical conviction suggests that the heating could be reduced when 30 cm-free spaces are interposed at least between two different secondary packages. The risk of chemical degradations and microbial spreading could be increased if plastic secondary boxes are used because of coefficients of thermal transmission for polymeric materials.

2.2.3 Operational Requirements

The continuous evolution of packaging and FP in particular is influenced by different needs, including 'new' usability requirements. At present, the possibility of using the original food container for heating, cooling or serving packaged foods becomes one of the fundamental and motivational elements for normal consumers. The profound change of current lifestyles has undoubtedly modified the consumeristic behaviour. The IFP should be easily handy and resealable [24]; in addition, it should be dimensionally reduced with possibility of little portions because of the important increase of single (individual) meals, the current 'fast food' tendency to shorter times and the diffusion of intuitive devices [25]. Designers can be extremely creative and produce innovative FP for futuristic IFP, but every new design needs adaptable materials (the role of synthetic chemistry is the first priority here) and good technologies for production, packaging, superficial treatment and storage.

Another reflection should be made with relation to environmental and sustainable policy statements. New functional requirements have been recently examined in last times: two examples are the need for improving dosing systems and 'durable' FP for repeated uses (the extension of shelf life does not concern the packaged food, but the exterior packaging). Moreover, the possible food contamination by 'Non-intentionally Added Substances' (NIAS) has recently highlighted the role of the recycling of packaging waste in the EU [26]. On the other side, European Institutions and national Agencies do not appear ready to give long-term answers to consumers at present [27, 28]. The most recent of these 'alarms' has concerned the detection of mineral oils in packaged foods and the possible risk on the human health; however, it has to be noted the European Food Safety Authority (EFSA) has clearly advised that safety risks by intake of mineral oils are not known or demonstrated [27].

2.2.4 Requirements for Packaging Disposal

The difficult management of packaging wastes is one of most important critical points in the modern world. With exclusive reference to the European situation, 78.4 million tonnes of packaging wastes are produced every year according to Eurostat [29]. This situation cannot be easily circumscribed to the simple and geographically well-defined portion of 'industrialised countries': other nations must face the menace of waste super-production without reliable disposal opportunities. Moreover, every possible solution should concern the whole life-cycle of FP and IFP instead of the simple last step of disposal. Consequently, a correct strategy should be planned in the design step.

As mentioned earlier, the possibility of toxic effects on human health is one of most important worries today. The problem has been recently correlated with FP when produced by recycled materials also. Additionally, the European regulatory has been enforced with the Regulation (EC) No 1907/2006 concerning the Registration, Evaluation, Authorisation and Restriction of Chemicals (REACH). This Regulation has clearly introduced new rules with reference to chemical substances, their identification and the authorisation or possible restrictions to the use for the production of industrial products in the EU. Naturally, only allowed chemicals can be used to produce FP in Europe. Moreover, the possible or sure recycling of 'long life' FP or other packaging wastes may introduce several of prohibited or 'suspected' substances [27].

Anyway, every disposal requirement for FP involves clearly materials, their chemical composition and the possibility of safe recycling from the functional angle. However, there are different recycling technologies and dissimilar materials; consequently, different recycling performances may be obtained with correlated impacts on the control of gaseous emissions, when measured as 'carbon footprint', and energy consumption [30, 31]. It should be also noted that recycling performances may be influenced by the peculiar connection between different FP components. For example, recyclable packages may be 'chemically' contaminated because of the use of peculiar glues or adhesive products of different origin [32, 33]. Another important factor is the possibility of reducing the encumbrance of recyclable FP.

On the other side, different components of similar FP may be painstakingly separated and recycled. For this and other reasons, FP designers should create new FP easy to disassemble: so the environmental impact of FP wastes may be reduced with similar strategies. On the other hand, the concept of easy separation between different components can represent a precise environmentally sustainable choice of food and non-food materials in peculiar 'poor' markets: the example of 'fair trade commerce' is notable, at present. Moreover, the lacking of raw material availability and reliable packing machineries in certain sites should be remembered. Substantially, the location of food productions in economically disadvantaged areas (with impetuous and often uncontrolled industrialisation) may impose difficult conditions.

The chronic deficiency of energy and transport infrastructures may also undermine certain food productions and stop economic investments [34]. As a result, the on-site production of basic and primary FP with minimal features becomes absolutely necessary: for example, paper and board packaging might be produced without glues, adhesive additives, printing inks, etc. Naturally, this situation has to be carefully examined when speaking of food packaging.

2.2.5 Communication Requirements

Original FP have been created with functional purposes (preservation and protection). Subsequent evolutions have determined in the '50s the transformation of FP into a communication media. As a result, the communication function of modern FP is considered as important as the functional one.

Actually, communication messages can be:

- Tacitly manipulated for mere commercial purposes with ethical implications, or
- Explicit with the aim of communicating positive ethical elements and environmentally sustainable features of the IFP (food and packaging are on the same ground).

With reference to communication, designers can choose between different requirements depending on the final goal [35].

In fact, FP has to direct the attention of the users to the related IFP despite the presence of different, but similar competitors. This is the 'appellative' function of packaging. In addition, FP must highlight the brand (identifying function) and direct the target to the desired object until the final choice (persuasive function). Finally, the FP should confirm consumers' expectations with adequate information about food product (informative function) and the effective communication of the main features (prescriptive function).

This theoretical dissertation should be chemically 'translated'. Following sections are dedicated to the detailed discussion of sub-requirements with the aim of demonstrating that:

- A generic FP may comply with different functions, and
- Industrial chemistry may supply (or be forced to give) suitable solutions for dissimilar objectives.

Before starting with this dissertation, it should be remembered that every design activity can bring advantages and disadvantages at the same time. In other words, FP can surely be excellent communication medium, but they can easily and rapidly communicate IFP failures at the same time, with dangerous effects.

2.2.5.1 Appellative Function

Generally, main sales channels are based on the so-called 'self service' system: every consumer buys products without intermediary services. Moreover, department stores can offer many food and non-food products with different brands, weights, volumes and prices. Naturally, FP have an important role: every IFP has to be immediately identified and recognised among other competitors [36, 37].

The concept of 'brand appellation' is not necessarily linked to FP: essential graphic elements may be useful and the use of thin colours can be a distinctive advantage when the attention of consumers has to be appealed without negative influence on persuasive functions. This communication effect can be easily reached in two different ways.

On the one side, FP may be completely transparent or minimally coloured (with a little percentage of covered printed areas). The aim is to show the inner content to interested consumers. For example designers can choose:

- Glass
- Flexible composite materials (closure: thermosealing option). Examples: metallised films for package snacks; flexible bags with a peelable seal covering a dedicated opening, for 1-stop shopping [15]
- 'Hybrid' packaging (the vision of edible content is partially allowed).

With reference to the last situation, it has to be noted the recent proposal of certain paper and board packaging with 'transparent' windows (naturally, every opening is protected with plastic films like polyethylene). Clearly, these choices—glass bottles and jars, composite and hybrid FP—are expressly fit for peculiar IFP categories and usable food packaging machinery. Moreover, the choice of raw materials (glass, paper and board, aluminium, adhesives, inks, flexible plastic films, etc.) can determine the success of IFP in terms of specific advantages (shelf life extension, better appearance, etc.) and opposite disadvantages (packaging ruptures, strange or grotesque colours, abnormal sensorial properties without clear hygiene concerns, etc.).

On the other side, designers may propose completely coloured and/or printed FP with the aim of projecting most known and inviting attributes of packaged foods. For example, metallic cans show usually external printed images with food representations: these pictures are normally 'better' than original foods because of the intrinsic brightness in contrast with the metallic nature of cans and the plastic composition of coatings and inks on can surfaces, depending also on the type of packaged product [10].

2.2.5.2 Identifying Function

As stated earlier, FP have to be easily correlated with the food category and a specific brand [1]. Generally, the identifying function should immediately comply with these requirements.

With reference to macro food categories, two factors have to be mainly considered:

- The final shape and the immediate appearance of the packaged product
- The composition of exterior FP (materials and components).

For example, the classical glass bottle is normally correlated with wines and other alcoholic beverages because of its own shape and the related composition (transparent glass). However, recent developments in the FP industry have generated new plastic bottles. The correlation between 'synthetic' packaging (the 'synthetic' term is naturally linked to plastic matters, while glass materials are perceived as traditional materials) and wines may appear difficult. In fact, European consumers are well-accustomed at least to associate intuitively traditional wines with traditional glass-made bottles.

On the other hand, the simple concept of plastic bottles is not based on the same and complex system of cultural and historical models if compared with traditional packaging for wines. Several wines are usually fermented in glass bottles instead of the most known barrel or *barrique* fermentation: consequently, glass is synonymous with tradition and wine technology for a notable part of consumers.

This example can be very useful because of strict relationships between original raw materials for FP production and the final use of food contact approved packaging. Basically, the normal consumer cannot be requested to know and/or study chemistry of polymers, glass systems, metals and so on. The food consumer is spontaneously able to classify packaged foods in spite of a certain and unavoidably simplistic approach. For example, the behaviour of modern consumers is easily predictable in front of classic 'tin cans': this FP typology is undoubtedly associated to a relatively short list of processed foods: vegetables, soups, peas, beans, tuna fish and meat products. The normal consequence is the automatic equation 'preserved food' = 'canned food' with the creation of a well-defined food category on the 'apparent' basis of the exterior FP.

On the other hand, tin cans are not easily associated with other non-processed foods (vegetable oils are a notable exception). Anyway, it has to be considered that the above-mentioned associations and classifications are mainly operated by consumers without solid knowledge of chemistry, microbiology, food technology and engineering: a very interesting result [36].

The correct identification of brands is strongly linked to the visual appearance of FP: printed logos, peculiar pictures and other graphic information in strict cooperation with the general aspect of the IFP and/or visible sensorial properties [38, 39]. It should be highlighted that this aspect: every known brand name is always connected with (a) pictorial images on FP and (b) physicochemical features of the complete IFP. With reference to the first point, the chromatic performance of certain glass jars is heavily influenced [5] by:

- The chemical composition of used labels
- The chemical composition of used dyes on labels and glass surfaces because of the influence on 'light solidity' of inks (the colorimetric resistance under light exposure)
- The chemical composition of coated supports (glass) because of the connection between chemical elements and brightness performance
- The physical appearance of jars in terms of rough or smooth surfaces (this feature is linked to processing technologies and finishing techniques)

Additionally, chemical features of the whole IFP are function of the exterior FP and the packaged food at the same time. For example, colorimetric performances of certain 'Maghreb' products such as *harissa* sauces in glass jars are dependent on the chemical composition of the edible content in synergy with the exterior container. In addition, the sensorial appearance of these products—*harissa* sauces may appear more or less 'red'—might be easily linked to some peculiar brand by consumers. This phenomenon may not be in connection with printed brands! The example of *harissa* sauces highlights the importance of more or less 'transparent' jars in certain situations.

2.2.5.3 Persuasive Function

Another important element is the so-called 'persuasive stimulus' on users. Once more, different factors have to be considered:

- Visual effects: colours, printed texts and images
- Synesthetic effects: shape, chemistry of materials and odours [5, 36, 37].

With reference to the above-shown features, the mention of chemistry of materials can be surprising. However, the simple introduction of printing inks may be useful to understand the penetration of industrial chemistry in such a case. The different chromatic performance of recent organic dyes and 'traditional' pigments can explain well the observable difference between opposite choices of consumers in front of two distinct, but similar IFP. The general strategy is based on the use of the most recognisable and bright tint, but other 'minimalist' approaches—simple colours, little chromatic tones—can be successful when the aim is to avoid consumers' disorientation [10].

The above-mentioned 'persuasive power' is mainly based on conceptual elements. Because of the marketing strategy and the peculiar food macro category, best communication strategies should be evocative: IFP have to be rationally perceived as 'good' or 'excellent' articles. Moreover, FP have to be considered— and rationally approved—as ergonomic devices. Generally, communication strategies comprehend both conceptual elements in different proportions with the exception of certain IFP categories.

2.2.5.4 Informative Function

Basically, food descriptions are useful after the final choice of IFP; however, the information may have some role when consumers evaluate the peculiar food and ponder negative and positive values.

Anyway, every description has one main goal: to give important and necessary advices about the correct use or interpretation of the purchased product (for example: dietary prescriptions and adaptability for certain recipes).

As a result, FP becomes a sort of information medium. Important descriptions and useful data can be subdivided in different categories:

1. Chemical and organoleptic features of packaged foods; shelf life; FP, when the description is mandatory; environmental sustainability; etc.
2. Advices for the correct use: opening, closure, dosing systems, peculiar warranties, useful phone numbers, etc.
3. Information for correct disposal.

Several advices are mandatory; other data are placed on FP because of their interest for particular consumeristic groups. Anyway, the non-redundant placement of information on the final IFP can determine the success [40].

Texts, images and icons have to be organised with the aim of helping the 'targeted' subject to understand the IFP [41, 42]. In other words, consumers have to be helped when remembering well-defined pictorial hierarchies and visual symbols. This reflection should clarify the role of information: should targets be peculiar people classes with cognitive specificity or physical deficiencies (children, elderlies, etc.), every possible stimulus—touch, sound, etc.—is equally useful and necessary [35].

In addition, several images can give different information with the arrival of new digital technologies and applications for mobile phones, tablets and modern Radio Frequency Identification (RFID) analysers. One of these innovations is currently represented by 'active' and 'intelligent packaging' devices: these instruments can allow the prompt and complete traceability of IFP lots with precious information about the qualitative state of packaged foods [14–43].

With exclusive relation to the chemical viewpoint, some reflection has to be obligatorily made.

First of all, the 'correct' placement of pictures—including related dimensions and reciprocal positions—may represent the concrete expression of a precise design strategy for the creation of the 'best' FP, depending on available productive models and materials. In other words, the availability of particular materials, intermediate chemicals and correlated production technologies can surely influence the dimension and other visible features of texts and images.

The formulation of printing inks and coatings may be very complex. For example, the following list shows a synthetic and non-exhaustive choice of pigments, resins and additives for food and non-food printing inks [44]:

- Inorganic pigments: titanium dioxide (white), carbon black (black), powdered aluminium (aluminated effect), 'Prussian blue' or $Fe_4[Fe(CN)_6]_3 \cdot xH2O$
- Organic pigments: azo pigments; beta-naphtol pigments; dioxazine pigments; quinophthalone; toluidine red—'International Union of Pure and Applied Chemistry ' (IUPAC) name, (1Z)-1-[(4-methyl-2-nitrophenyl) hydrazinylidene] naphthalen-2-one
- Mineral fillers: kaolin types
- Optical brightener agents
- Photoinitiators like isopropyl thioxanthone, also named ITX
- Plasticisers
- Waxes
- Wetting agents
- Binders: rosin resins, maleic resins and alkyd resins
- Solvents and diluents: mineral oils, fatty acid esters and vegetable oils (soy bean oil, linseed oil, etc.)
- Siccative agents, also known as drying accelerators for oil coatings (alkyd resins) and printing inks: cobalt and cobalt-free carboxylates. For cobalt-free compounds, manganese and iron appear good options.

The choice of best pigments or coatings depends on metallic supports (with relation to the presence of aesthetical failures) and the possible presence of 'strange' colorimetric features of the packaged product. For example, the known 'ghosting effect'—the appearance of 'negative' pictures on inner surfaces of metal cans, while 'positive' images are printed on external surfaces—can be avoided [36] by:

1. Augment of polymerisation temperatures into ovens,
2. Increase of polymerisation times into ovens,
3. Use of different printing inks without affinity for inner coatings.

Secondly, digital technology seems to have displayed new options when speaking of relations between FP users and IFP consumers. At present, FP failures, including future imperfections because of different causes, can be detected and examined easily by means of image analysis software. Similar studies have already been carried out in different fields like chemistry of conservation and restorations.

With exclusive reference to food packaging analyses in the EU, the main goal should be to define and develop reliable procedures for rapid FP controls. Should these systems be created and used by FM, the correct and mandatory 'assessment of technological suitability to the intended use' for FP would be easy, economically convenient and demonstrable without complex analytical protocols [10].

2.2.6 Environmental Requirements

At present, environmental sustainability is extremely debated in different fields. One of major concerns is the problem of packaging wastes [26, 45, 46]: this important issue cannot be solved with recycling activities despite notable improvements in recent years from the regulatory and the technological views. In fact, packaging design has been progressively oriented to environmental topics: useful demonstrations are the study of 'green' materials and the concomitant reduction of volumetric capacities and consumed energy in the 'carbon footprint' perspective. However, more efforts are still needed.

The simple quantitative approach to the problem of FP wastes may 'mask' other qualitative critical points: the uneasy separation of joint components and the consequent 'contamination' of mono-material recycled materials; the wide use of composite packages ('hybrid' packaging without a well-defined material classification), the presence of materials difficult to identify etc. As a result, the final performance or 'yield' of industrial recycling—the ratio between the quantity of reusable matter and the initial waste—cannot reach 100 % [34].

For these reasons, the maximisation of material recycling may be obtained if qualitative and quantitative factors are taken into account in the design step. However, environmental requirements have to be satisfied with productive and marketing needs [47], including also the clear separation between food macro-categories and related chemical concerns (different contamination episodes etc.).

It has to be noted that FP environmental requirements do not constitute a single category without other connections: the environmental defence involves different aspects [48, 49], including FPM recycling: on this level all packaging requirements have to be considered.

2.2.7 Regulatory Requirements

Regulatory requests have to be carefully considered when speaking of packaging design. The complete and exhaustive analysis of the regulatory situation in different macroeconomic areas should be highly recommended: however, this discussion is not the basic aim of this book. On the other hand, it may be displayed here a brief and synthetic description of the current EU regulatory concerning FPM.

Existing EU Regulations, norms, voluntary standards and protocols may influence designers' choices: at the same time, chemical features of FP and IFP are dependent on mandatory requirements because of different factors including food safety also. With exclusive reference to FP and features of single materials, the interested reader is invited to consult more specific references.

With relation to EU countries, two regulatory protocols have notable influence on the work of FP designers. By the chemical viewpoint, main requests can be summarised as follows.

First of all, every packaging material for food contact applications has to comply with the Regulation (EC) No 2023/2006 with concern to the obligatory implementation of a system of 'Good Manufacturing Practices' (GMP) by FP producers, distributors and industrial users of FPM and FP. This approach should assure the 'quality' of food contact approved materials and give adequate warranties about the control of the above-defined quality.

In other words, all FP have to be compliant with all applicable norms and defined quality standards with express reference to the intended final use. Anyway, FP is not allowed to cause risks to human health and modify the composition of packaged products with consequent unacceptable failures, including every variation of organoleptic features. It has to be noted that variations are always referred to packaged foods instead of the whole IFP. However, it should be also remembered that all possible damages or modifications of FP can affect the qualitative and quantitative composition of packaged products.

Another important document, the Regulation (EC) No 1935/2004, concerns basic features of food contact approvable materials.

In detail, FP have to be compliant with existing GMP; consequently, they cannot transfer excessive amounts of foreign components to packaged foods in normal and predictable conditions. The final aim is to avoid that contaminated foods may (a) be harmful for the human health and (b) determine unacceptable modifications of food products with reference to composition and sensorial features. Naturally, the chemical composition is inextricably connected to organoleptic features: every little chemical modification may be easily recognised by means of simple sensorial testing methods.

An interesting example concerns processed or analogue cheeses. These products are normally packaged in thermosealable and flexible FP. At first, packaging materials are sold, delivered and stored near FM as simple spools. As a result, the final shape and aspect of packaged cheeses are different from the initial shape of FP before use.

For this reason, the detection of sensorial failures may be easily carried out by operators before use. This obligation is named 'evaluation of technological suitability' in the EU [5]. However, food operators should know or be aware of FP possible failures and complications because of incorrect storage conditions, for example. As a result, it may be assumed that the above-mentioned cheeses may show abnormal colours on surfaces because of the emersion or visible appearance of red spots. Actually, this phenomenon may have distinct causes:

- Food contact transfer of red colorants (printing inks) from the external surface of FP to the inner surface of spools (this situation is known as 'ghosting' effect) and subsequent migration of red inks on food surfaces
- Chemical modification of superficial colours by microbial spreading.

The first cause is clearly dependent on FP. However, the simple storage in incorrect conditions of spools—high temperature and light exposure—can easily worsen observable defects. Similar failures may be easily discovered before use.

The second situation is dependent on microbial spreading. Generally, one of credible causes is the abundant production of red pigments like prodigiosin: molecular formula: $C_{20}H_{25}N_3O$, IUPAC name: (2Z,5Z)-3-methoxy-2-[(5-methyl-4-pentyl-1H-pyrrol-2-yl) methylidene]-5-pyrrol-2-ylidenepyrrole. This pigment is produced by coliform bacteria like *Serratia marcescens* [50].

The occurrence of such a similar contamination can be attributed to simple FP environmental contamination by means of aerosolised dispersions into food production plants. However, the possibility of cheese contamination is initially taken into account [51].

In addition, packaged cheeses show often other interesting and unpleasant features: the augment of moisture is generally concomitant with the weak decrease of fat content values [51, 52] and the notable diminution of proteins. The subsequent production of sulphur amino acids, simple hydrogen sulphide and low molecular weight (MW) molecules by casein decomposition is correlated with (a) excessive cheese softness and (b) negative oxidation-reduction potentials. Basically, these conditions are caused by microbial spreading (coliforms, other lactose-fermenting bacteria and proteolytic micro organisms). However, it should be noted that high environmental humidity can cause the same problem when stored FP are quite able to absorb aqueous vapours on surfaces. This situation highlights the importance of good manufacturing practices in FPP and food production plants also.

Regulation (EC) No 1935/2004 considers all possible FP, including 'active' (also named 'smart') and 'intelligent' objects and materials (Sect. 2.2.1) [14]. Actually, the complete regulatory panorama is extremely complex and in continuous evolution: as a consequence, a single FP or packaging component should be examined on the basis of the above-mentioned Regulations and other national and EU protocols concerning other important aspects of IFP and FP (examples: nutritional labelling, restrictions of use for peculiar materials according to REACH legislation etc.). The interested reader is invited to consult more specific references.

Additionally, there are also specific and 'voluntary' protocols with relation to quality systems, food safety, environmental management, etc. At present, food safety and quality assurance are jointly managed according to most recognised quality standards:

- The ISO 22000:2005 norm by the International Organisation for Standardization (ISO)
- The Global Standard for Food Safety (GSFS) by the British Retail Consortium (BRC)

- The International Featured Standard (IFS) Food, by the IFS
- The 'Food Safety System Certification' (FSSC):22000 by the Foundation for Food Safety Certification.

With reference to FP, other voluntary norms have been recently created: the most known of these protocols is the 'BRC/IOP Global Standard for Packaging and Packaging Materials' by the BRC and the Packaging Society, formerly known as the Institute of Packaging (IoP).

All the above-mentioned standards are completely voluntary. However, FM or FPP cannot supply main mass retailer groups without one or more of related certifications. As a clear consequence, FP designers have to comply with 'voluntary' requirements also, in spite of their unmandatory nature [5].

2.2.8 Food Packaging Materials: Composition, Production, Chemical Features and Correlations with Packaging Design

This Section is dedicated to FP from the viewpoint of chemistry. Actually, the chemical composition of raw materials, intermediates and finished packages can influence and/ or be influenced by designers' choices. In particular, the group of functional requirements is strongly linked to the chemistry and the technology of FP and final IFP. As a result, the careful examination of FP should be recommended and possibly correlated with functional requirements.

First of all, the classification of FP has to be made on the basis of a few parameters. Normally, two approaches may be tried:

- FP can be classified on the basis of the used raw materials and the final appearance [53]
- On the other hand, FP may be classified depending on the final use or food destination [5, 54].

The first approach has been chosen with reference to this book because many of possible advantages and failures for FP are dependent from the chemical nature of non-edible materials. After all, one peculiar food can be packaged with 'n' different packages: as a result, 'n' different behaviours may be expected depending on the peculiar container. Every FP category can be now discussed in relation to:

- Simplified subcategories of food containers or separated components
- Used raw materials
- The simplified description of FP structures
- Advantages and possible failures of final IFP
- Correlations with functional requisites.

2.2.8.1 Metal Packages

The well known 'tin can' is simply the first and most recognisable subtype of metal container for food applications [5, 36].

Actually, the first mention should be made with exclusive reference to key properties of original raw materials [54]. As a consequence, metal containers have following positive features:

- Notable rigidity and tensile strength
- Excellent 'barrier effect' against light, other external agents and penetrating fluids or solids
- High density for steel-made FP
- Low density for aluminium-made FP

By contrast, these containers cannot be sealed without adequate plastic or metallic closures. In addition, metallic and plastic raw materials can interact with edible foods [54]. These basic features depend mainly on the composition of basic supports: steel or aluminium.

Steel Supports

Basically, steel materials can be found on the market of metal containers in different forms, depending on the peculiar composition and protection processes against the metallic corrosion. Generally, three materials are fully recognisable at present.

Electrolytic Tin Plate (ETP) is a low-carbon steel with a thin superficial coating. This protection is obtained by the electrolytic deposition of metallic tin on the surface of black carbon steel coils. The structure of ETP is complex enough. With the exclusion of the steel support, following layers may be observed [36]:

- Intermetallic iron-tin complex ($FeSn_2$), with approximate thickness of 10^{-4} mm
- Metallic tin, approximate thickness: 10^{-3} mm
- Mixed oxides of tin and chromium: SnO_2, SnO, CrO_3; approximate thickness: 10^{-4} mm
- Calcium carbonate (from normal washing treatments), variable thickness
- And finally an organic layer such as dioctyl sebacate (DOS) against the superficial oxidation.

It should be noted that DOS and similar 'protections' cannot prevent chemical interactions between food products and non-coated metal surfaces. For this reason, steel-made packages are usually coated with organic resins and enamels with the aim of avoiding the direct contact between tin surfaces and 'attacking' foods such as white fruits and tomato-based products [54]. Another good support is Tin Free Steel (TFS), also named 'Electrolytic Chromium oxide Coated Steel' (ECCS). With relation to this material, the original low carbon-steel coil is electrolytically coated with a superficial layer of chrome/chrome oxide [54]. This material needs also an organic protection against the superficial corrosion.

Other possible materials could be 'black plates' or 'coke' tinplates. However, their use has to be carefully considered because black surfaces of uncoated steel plates are easily attacked by environmental oxygen and moisture. With reference to 'coke' materials, these supports correspond to the 'old' version of ETP materials: the deposition of metallic tin is highly irregular. Consequently, adhesion problems may occur when these materials are coated with organic resins or enamels [36].

Aluminium Supports

The first subcategory of metal containers is recognised as 'steel-made' FP because of the use of coated or uncoated steel supports. By contrast, the second subclass of metal cans is identified as 'aluminium-made' FP because of the use of aluminium alloys. It has to be noted that peculiar features of these materials (ductility and low density) determine the final destination of FP.

Chemically, it can be affirmed that aluminium 'alloys' contain also manganese, magnesium and other metals in very low proportions. Normally, mechanical performances can be modified with the addition of non-aluminium metals, magnesium and manganese above all [54]. Another interesting property of aluminium alloys is the impossibility of welding processes differently from ETP; actually, ECCS also cannot be welded. Consequently, aluminium-made containers are generally defined as 'two-piece' FP because of the subdivision of the structure in a basic body and one mechanically-sealed end. On the other hand, steel-made containers can be produced as 'three-piece' metal cans (one body and two ends), 'two-piece' single drawn, multiple drawn, and drawn and wall ironed cans [5, 36, 54].

It should be added that aluminium-made containers are necessarily coated with organic coatings on the inner (food-contact) side for preventing damages to metallic surfaces by foods.

Simplified Description of Metal Containers

It can be also assumed that the description of metal containers is difficult enough: many subtypes of steel-made FP are possible, and the same thing can be affirmed when speaking of aluminium cans. However, a simplified description can be given when speaking of the 'old' three-piece metal can. This steel-made container has the following features [5, 54]:

- The external appearance of the packaging is determined by the presence of a single 'body' with a cylindrical shape. This cylinder is obtained by the welding on two different sides of the same steel sheet. For this reason, ETP materials may be used while TFS/ECCS or aluminium supports cannot be considered

- Two different but similar 'can ends' are applied on the body with the aim of assuring the complete sealability and the protection of contained foods against external agents. The junction is mechanically assisted without welding. For this reason, a thin layer of organic product (polyvinyl chloride gaskets or similar products) is interposed between body and end surfaces because the simple mechanical junction may be insufficient for hermetical closures
- Can ends are normally available as regular or easy-open ends, depending on the specific need and requests of FM. Easy-open ends are also known as 'stay-on tab' systems. The last of these ends is specifically designed for drink (aluminium) cans [54]
- Generally, external and inner sides of body and ends are coated with organic lacquers or enamels. Several exceptions may be tolerated when speaking of non-aggressive foods (examples: weak acid fluids). On the other side, acid or high-pigmented foods such as *harissa* sauces may easily attack metallic surfaces with the consequent corrosion and the dissolution of metallic ions into foods and FP damages. In addition, the external appearance of 'tin cans' is decorated with lithographic systems (Sect. 5.1.2). With the exclusion of two-piece drawn and wall-ironed containers, coating and lithographic operations are made on flat, coil or sheet metal supports. Every coating, enamel and printing ink has to be cured into conventional ovens or under UV lamps: the curing process implies the polymerisation of pre-polymerised resins.

Metal Packages: Advantages and Possible Failures of the Final Product

Many metal containers seem to define a peculiar class of preserved foods. In detail, the description 'canned food' means a diversified but well known miscellany of IFP. The following list is not exhaustive, but several of the most important 'canned' products are mentioned here:

- Canned fish
- Preserved vegetables (peas, maize, beans, …)
- Vegetable oils

With relation to canned foods, following advantages should be always taken into account:

- Easy preservation, depending on the peculiar preservation during and after the packaging
- Low storage temperatures are not strictly required
- The final IFP is extremely resistant against mechanical damages during transportation and storage steps
- The presence of reduced air into packaged foods is one of main requirements for acceptable closures. As a result, it may be assumed that 'regular' canned foods should not suffer problems by air oxidation

- Finally, thermal treatments (pasteurisation, sterilisation etc.) require that used FP may be resistant enough to sudden temperature leaps. This feature may be a problem when using certain FP, but metal containers should comply with this important requisite. In addition, metal cans may be also used as cooking, self-heating or self-cooling instruments [5].

On the other side, different problems and failures can occur. Actually, defects of the final IFP may be seen as the 'other side' of metal containers because of the insufficient, defective or lacking performance of FP and/or foods. Anyway, it may be assumed that the most part of all known features are related to the chemistry of metal FP, their intermediates and food products.

The following list shows most known defects of canned foods with a chemical origin and the related explanation [5, 36, 54].

Corrosion of Metal Supports and Dissolution of Metallic Ions into Foods

The detection of iron, tin, chromium, copper ions or other foreign metals into certain acid foods (hot sauces etc.) or preserved fruit juices is caused by:

- Insufficient coating of metal surfaces by organic lacquers or enamels, and/or
- Presence of micro or macro bubbles into organic coatings or enamels, and/or
- Presence of micro scratches on coated surfaces.

Anyway, four results can be observed: (1) the attack of uncoated metal surfaces by organic acids or pigments from foods; (2) the detection of metallic ions into foods; (3) the dissolution of inorganic elements from demolished white enamels when used (many metallic FP are white-coated on the inner side; white enamels contain usually titanium oxide) and finally (4) the partial demolition of organic networks (lacquers, enamels) with the possible detection of suspect intermediates.

The fundamental role of tin as a sacrificial anode in the corrosion process should be highlighted. However, this process is not rapid because of the superficial presence of hydrogen. In addition, superficial iron would be demolished by food products without tin protection with chromatic alterations, off-flavours and can swelling [54]. Anyway, critical factors for the dissolution of tin are generally: storage temperatures, the extension of uncovered areas, insufficient coating thickness, excessive amount of residual oxygen, passivation, high acidity and notable quantities of organic pigments in certain products. The possible presence of 'catalysing' ions such as nitrate should be also remembered [54].

Other contaminants may cause notable worries [5, 54]. The dissolution of iron may cause colorimetric modifications in peculiar foods. Aluminium could cause cloudiness or haze in sensitive beverages (beers). Sulphur staining (blue-black or brown marks on the inner side of coated ETP- or TFS- cans) is well known. The critical factor is the presence of foods with notable protein amounts (peas and fish). In fact, the attack of hydrogen sulphide (H_2S) to coated tin surfaces causes the formation of iron sulphides, oxides and hydroxides (black or brown substances). Normally, the solution is offered by 'zinc oxide' (ZnO) paste: this fluid material is produced with epoxyphenolic resins and added to organic coatings for food-contact side. The reaction between H_2S and metallic surfaces produces white zinc sulphide instead of black substances. However, the defect may be important depending on the quantity of added ZnO paste. Moreover, the occurrence of white or black colours is important because of the demonstration of the chemical permeability of epoxyphenolic coatings with relation to acid attacks.

Corrosion of Metal Supports and Other Failures

The corrosion of metal supports can be cause of different failures. One of most discussed dangers in recent years has been the detection of bisphenol A and other chemicals (intermediates in the production of selected organic resins) such as bisphenol A diglycidyl ether in foods [5, 54]. In fact, organic lacquers are generally produced and used as dispersions of selected pre-polymerised matters: epoxyphenolic, epoxidic, polyester, vinyl resins etc. These coatings are usually deposed on metallic surfaces and cured at different temperatures into dedicated ovens. For example, a general epoxyphenolic coating may be completely polymerised on metal surfaces after 15 min at 200 °C, with the exclusion of UV lacquers [55]. Superficial organic layers are very thin (up to 15 μm), but several differences might be observed. Anyway, every can coating, enamel or similar product should assure [5]:

- Good resistance to thermal treatments (sterilisation, pasteurisation etc.)
- Good mechanical resistance to impacts, drawing and stretching
- Excellent chemical inertness
- Absence or reduction of food adhesiveness (packaged foods may adhere to organic surfaces such as canned salmon in polyester-coated cans).

Anyway, the detection of organic intermediates in foods may have following causes [5]:

- Superficial fractures, presence of damaged micro bubbles (also named 'blistering' effect)
- Incomplete reticulation (polymerisation) of pre-polymerised resins on metal surfaces
- Rheological instability of liquid coatings, including storage failures
- Partially active fractions of organic resins and/or inks. Ink residues may be transferred from the external to the inner side of cans because of the simple contact between unassembled sheets. This defect is named 'ghosting'
- Insufficient adhesion of coatings to metallic surfaces (low chromium amounts mean low chelating effects).

Other can failures without direct food safety consequences concern the external side: once more, origins are related to chemistry and process controls [5]:

- Chemical incompatibility between enamels and printing inks
- Chemical incompatibility between inks and the finishing or transparent coating

- Superposition of different inks on the same zone
- Excessive water quantity (printing inks are hydrophobic)
- Presence of micro water bubbles in the printed area after sterilisation (also named 'meshing' effect).

2.2.8.2 Glass Packages

Glass bottles, jars and similar containers have a long historical tradition [56].

From a general viewpoint, glass is a versatile material for food and non-food applications. Normally, following properties are well known and recognisable when speaking of similar containers [53, 56]:

- Chemical inertness
- Impermeability
- Transparency
- Rigidity
- Breakability
- Virtual endless reusability
- Superficial properties (smooth appearance, roughened ice-like effect etc.)
- Different shapes
- Perceived hygiene

By contrast, glass packages are surely fragile and are not usually closed with glass systems because of the insufficient hermeticity. Mentioned features depend strongly on the peculiar chemical composition and possible differences on the market. Moreover, the importance of recycled materials cannot be excluded: 50 % and more of the total amount of raw materials for glass containers are recycled at present.

Chemical Composition of Glass Materials

It may be affirmed that glass corresponds to a melted mixture of silica, lime and soda materials [56]. The result of the fusion may be defined as a metastable system: the ordered glass network is continually 'blocked' in one of the possible high-energy viscous structures, from the thermodynamic viewpoint. By contrast, the most preferred structure should be highly chaotic and fluid.

Five main typologies of glass materials may be recognised at present [56]:

- White flint (or clear) glass
- Dark green glass
- Pale green glass
- Blue glass
- Amber glass

White Flint Glass

Basically, 'clear' glass corresponds [56] to the 'pure' melted mixture of silica (72 %), lime or calcium oxide (12 %) and soda or sodium oxide (12 %). Other minerals may be present depending on the composition of original raw materials: alumina, magnesium oxide and potassium oxide. The 'neutral' appearance is function of the absence of chromatically recognisable mineral elements with distinct colours. In other words, the 'white' and completely transparent glass corresponds to a tri-dimensional matrix based on silicon, oxygen, sodium and calcium. This network contains many intra-molecular empty spaces, also named 'vacancies', with the possible addition of different metallic ions. Should vacancies be filled with a metallic cation, the macroscopic network should appear as a coloured and possibly transparent matter to an external observer. The absence of recognisable colours is function of silicon, sodium and calcium.

Dark Green Glass

This material is obtained [56] by means of the addition of chromium oxide (Cr_2O_3) and iron oxide (Fe_2O_3) to glass mixtures. Chemically, empty spaces are filled with chromium and iron: the result is the 'dark green' appearance of the network. Actually, the intensity of blue-green colours is mainly caused by the prevailing amount of trivalent chromium if compared with iron.

Pale Green Glass

This material, also named 'half white' glass, is obtained by means of the addition of Fe_2O_3 and Cr_2O_3 with the abundance of iron (green colour) if compared to trivalent chromium [56].

Blue Glass

Normal 'blue glass' can be obtained by means of the addition of cobalt ions to glass mixtures with low abundance of iron [56]. It should be considered that 'blue' types are very expensive in certain productions: as a clear result, blue bottles for carbonated soft drinks or mineral bottles may be expensive. The same thing can be told for the final IFP. For this reason, the chromaticity of certain beverages may be discussed with the aim of obtaining the desired colour of bottled products with transparent containers (Sect. 4.3.1).

Amber Glass

The last type of glass material is widely used in the market of light-sensitive beverages because of the 'filtering' function against UV rays (Sect. 4.3.1). The brown aspect of related bottles can be obtained by means of the addition of ferric ions to glass mixtures: ferrous ions should be much reduced [56]. In addition, carbon atoms are inserted in the tri-dimensional matrix, while chromium should be virtually absent [57].

Simplified Description of Glass Containers

Glass containers for food applications are generally subdivided in two categories [5]: bottles (for wines, beers, mineral waters etc.) and jars. Actually, different types and subtypes of glass FP can be designed. However, the most part of similar containers are often found in these two groups.

Anyway, the basic concept is not strictly related to the chemical composition of mineral mixtures. On the contrary, the shape of final containers is often determined after the evaluation of different factors [56]:

- Type of food product
- Volumetric capacity
- Type of closure (metallic or plastic system)
- Dimension of necks
- Typology of the filling process. Beverages and fluid foods may be hot-filled with possibility of pasteurisation, sterilisation, mixes systems, etc.
- Mechanic resistance of filled containers when piled up into pallets
- Necessity of UV protection for packaged foods.

With reference to bottles and jars, the description of forming procedures ('press and blow', 'blow and blow', and 'narrow neck press and blow' processes) may be not interesting when speaking of pure design and relations with chemical features of FP and IFP. On the contrary, surface treatments can be discussed.

In detail, the 'hot-end treatment' is designed [56] to prevent superficial damages on hot bottles (at the end of forming procedures). As a result, the strength of containers should be improved. Generally, tin oxide is used as coating; lubricant additives should be also used because of friction risks.

Alternatively, the 'cold-end treatment' may be used on annealed containers (residual strain has been removed). In detail, glass surfaces are lubricated with the addition of polyethylene, waxes etc. [56]. The discussion of this system can be important because several adhesive labels may not adhere properly to treated surfaces in spite of the presence of adequate dextrine products as adhesives.

Another important discussion should be made with concern to closures. At present, plastic or metallic caps are used for the most part of bottles despite the presence of common cork closures for wines [56]. Normally, following solutions are available:

- Tight fitting plugs
- Screw threaded caps
- Metal caps.

Other closures are possible with excellent results with relation to hermeticity [56]. Anyway, available closures are defined 'normal', 'vacuum' or 'pressure' seals depending on the peculiar system and the type of packaged product.

Glass Packages: Advantages and Possible Failures of the Final IFP

With relation to recognised advantages, glass materials have been already discussed. Generally, following properties are considered with positive results in the food sector [56]:

- Chemical inertness
- Impermeability
- Transparency
- Rigidity
- Breakability
- Virtual endless reusability
- Superficial properties
- Different shapes
- Perceived hygiene
- Retention to carbonated drinks.

In addition, the possibility of different printing techniques and labelling choices should be highlighted. On the other hand, possible failures of glass FP should be discussed with relation to the safety and integrity of the final IFP [5]. In detail, the following situations should be considered [5, 56, 57]:

- Superficial defects, including foreign bodies. Examples: micro 'stones'. Detection by means of scanning electron microscopy and X-ray microanalysis
- Micro bubbling. Detection by means of optical microscopy
- Micro fractures
- Scratches (forming and glass annealing procedures)
- Colorimetric variations. Detection by means of optical microscopy
- Insufficient UV protection (for light-sensitive foods)
- Mechanical damages (insufficient strength)
- Insufficient adhesion (when self-adhesive labels are used), including also the presence of condensate on glass surfaces
- Closure failures
- Defects by washing treatments
- Gradient failures
- Sharp edges, scraps and shivers
- Weathering of the inner surface (during storage, usually for white flint glass)
- Insufficient cleanliness, when speaking of reusable FP.

In particular:

- For micro bubbling, the total elimination of air bubbles in glass matrices should be obtained with the 'gradient' prolongation of melting procedures. Otherwise, micro air bubbles may 'force' glass structures to exhibit crystalline-like behaviours and thermodynamically-favoured amorphous structures. After all, containers can suffer possible fractures where micro bubbles are present

- With relation to colorimetric variations, this failure can be important for two reasons. First of all, many preserved foods are requested to exhibit uniform colours. This requirement should imply that transparent (coloured or 'white') glass jars show a defined and constant colorimetric tint, where expected [5]. However, the presence of different atoms with small amounts (iron, chromium etc.) has to be evaluated when speaking of normal jars by recycled glass materials. Because of the abundance of recycled matters, chromatic modifications of glass containers should be expected and possibly minimised, similarly to 'stones' and micro bubbles. These defects are virtually detectable in all possible glass containers. For these reasons, the use of optical microscopy and digital imaging techniques for the analysis of colours [10] can be very useful. In addition, colorimetric variations may damage several light-sensitive foods (insufficient UV protection) with clear worries for food packagers and producers
- The so-called 'weathering' of glass FP may be very important in the food sector because of the necessity of avoiding food contacts with abnormal surfaces. In detail, weathered surfaces of soda-lime silicate glasses show irregular white deposits of sodium and calcium carbonates [58]. The defect may be avoided or limited if environmental conditions are monitored with reference to the relative humidity. Generally, the best strategy for the examination of incorrectly stored glass materials is the visual evaluation, while other most sensitive procedures (electron microscopy, adsorption of generated alkali) appear useful for research purposes [59]
- The problem of the insufficient adhesion (with self-adhesive labels) is mainly caused by the presence of condensate on glass surfaces. Normally, glass has to be conditioned thermally to prevent this situation. However, 'cold end' containers show lubricated glass surfaces with the use of water-based polyethylene emulsions, derivatives of polyester waxes, etc. [56]. Actually, other substances might be used: soaps, stearates, silicones, glycerides, oleic acid, etc. However, their use is very limited or rejected by FM. For example, breweries should not accept oleic acid as lubricant for glassware in spite of the easy removability and low lubricant properties during storage periods, because of the possible flavour alteration of beers [60]. As a result, several adhesive labels may not adhere properly to treated surfaces. For this reason, new types of self adhesive labels may be designed for specific purposes: the formulation of adhesive products should contrast lubricating effects. Normally, casein adhesives are used extensively [61], but other solutions may be applied when high water resistance is required to labels for high speed processes [62]. Anyway, the problem can be also linked to the correct cold-end treatment: for instance, the use of water-base polyethylene emulsions requires the additional use of normal or distilled water. With the exception of nonionic polyethylene coating materials, the presence of calcium salts may affect the process and alter subsequent steps, including the choice and the adhesion of dedicated labels.

Glass Packages: Correlations with Functional Requisites

The good preservation and protection of foods in glass packages are strictly linked to the chemical inertness, the full or modified transparency and other variables: possible UV protection, impermeability to gases and vapours, rigidity and reusability [56].

Naturally, the inertness should be always assured: on the other side, several contaminations by alkali production (during the storage) and/or lubricant additives should be considered. However, the lubrication is absolutely needed for preventing superficial damages.

The transparency of glass containers is clearly expected by normal consumers: as a result, this requirement should be 'obvious'. Once more, superficial damages or weathering may cause important worries. In addition, the absence of peculiar colours (and the consequent UV protection of bottled beverages) may be seen as a distinctive advantage by the marketing viewpoint (Sect. 4.3.1) despite the number of available examples of glass FP with blue, amber and other colours [56].

Transportation and storage requirements are extremely important in the sector of glass containers and bottled beverages. For instance, beers and wines may require low storage temperatures. As a result, the final IFP must resist at least to the inner dilatation, the pressure of carbonated products and sudden bumps. In addition, the superficial appearance and the resistance to scratches have to be always assured.

With concern to operational requirements, glass containers may be used for 'ageing' packaged foods. This is not specifically true for preserved vegetables, sauces, seafood products and so on. On the other hand, red and some white wines can be initially aged in oak wood barrels and subsequently continue the ageing period in bottles for one or 2 years [63]. As a consequence, glass bottles can have a precise technological function with relation to the evolution of anthocyanins and non-anthocyanin phenolic compounds [64]. Naturally, the hermetic closure of bottles and the well known inertness of glass surfaces are important. In addition, glass packages are well recognised as resealable containers.

Finally, glass packages are reusable—the 'old' British example of fresh milk in reused bottles is well known—and easily recyclable with excellent results [56].

2.2.8.3 Plastic Packages

Plastic materials are used for the manufacturing of different food and non-food packages. With reference to food and beverage products, there are many possible solutions including also 'hybrid' packages: after all, the whole group of metal containers can be defined as the classic example of plastic/metallic container because of the synergic coexistence of metal supports and plastic coatings, enamels, gaskets and other organic components, including printing inks [54].

Probably, the classification of plastic packages may be very difficult because of two reasons:

– Every food or beverage may be associated with different packages, and
– The same plastic package may be designed and redeveloped with the aim of obtaining similar performances with different food products.

As a consequence, the best strategy could be the subdivision of the whole range of plastic FP in four macro categories without a direct food correlation. According to this approach [5], plastic packages for food applications may be classified and described as follows:

• Rigid and semirigid containers
• Flexible FP
• Polycoupled FP (these containers are different from flexible containers and plastic components)
• Plastic components for plastic and hybrid packages.

Rigid and Semirigid Plastic Containers

This macro category contains many typologies of plastic FP with peculiar features and different destinations. Generally, rigid plastic containers are produced [65] as:

• Bottles and jars (main competitor for this type of FP: glass packages)
• Trays and boxes
• Drums, intermediate bulk containers, crates, etc.
• Expanded or foamed plastic containers.

The rigidity of these containers may be strengthened or diminished depending on the composition of plastic mixtures. Normally, semirigid containers contain different polymeric materials and several additives with the aim of enlarging the possible range of plastic containers: economic reasons are certainly important, but other factors can be part of the final decision, including packaging disposal requirements.

Flexible Plastic Packages

This heterogeneous subgroup of plastic FP comprehends [5, 65]:

• Flexible heat-sealed bags, pouches and sachets
• Flexible films with possibility of heat sealability near FP
• Plastic films for wrapping and similar uses. Example: regenerated cellulose films.

This nonexhaustive list contains different types of plastic matters. Once more, plastic components and polymers may be mixed or coupled (example: coextruded plastic films) with the aim of obtaining enhanced strength, impermeability to vapours or gases, etc.

Polycoupled Food Packages

The class of polycoupled FP is continually evolving: in fact, the most part of new designs and redevelopments may be found in this subsector of the plastic industry.
    Generally, following types are found in this category [5, 65]:

- Polycoupled packages (plastic films and paperboard foils are joint)
- 'Tetrahedral' package systems (plastic films, aluminium and/or paperboard foils are joint).

This classification is very simplified: however, the aim of this book is to give evidence of correlations between the design of FP and physicochemical features of containers and final IFP. The interested reader is invited to consult more specific references.

Plastic Components for Plastic and Hybrid Packages

Finally, the group of plastic components for a whole range of plastic and 'hybrid' applications is mentioned. Actually, the below shown classification should also take into account the notable class of intermediate plastic films for coupling purposes. Following components may be mentioned [5, 36, 64]:

- Plastic lacquers, enamels, gaskets and printing inks for metal containers
- Plastic lids and caps (for closures)
- Plastic seals
- Dispensing systems
- Adhesive films, labels, etc.

Once more, the composition of these accessories can be diversified. In addition, there are not reasonable connections between the shape or other visible features of separated components and the chemical composition, with some exception. In fact, many factors—economic convenience, logistics, environmental policies, commercial requirements, etc.—should be considered; anyway, the final destination of FP has to be considered first.

On these bases, the discussion should now consider main plastic materials for food packaging applications. It can be anticipated that chemical features of polymers and plastic additives may heavily influence the design of a specified food packaging, although a whole range of intermediate possibilities and 'compromises' between different requests may be obtained.

Main Plastic Polymers

At present, the use of polymers for FP applications is mainly oriented to following chemicals [5, 36, 64]:

- Polyethylene (PE), also defined as 'low density polyethylene (LDPE), 'high density polyethylene' (HDPE). Other types are available
- Polypropylene (PP). Different varieties are available, including oriented polypropylene (OPP)
- Polystyrene (PS), including also expanded polystyrene (EPS)
- Polyvinyl chloride (PVC)
- Polyesters: polyethylene terephthalate (PET or PETE) and other varieties
- Polyvinylidene chloride (PVDC)
- Polyamides (PA)
- Ethylene vinyl acetate (EVA)
- Various ionomeric materials
- Ethylene vinyl alcohol (EVOH)
- Fluoropolymers
- Derivatives of cellulose.

This list cannot be exhaustive because of the complexity of the market of plastic matters [5]. After all, the most part of polymers for FP production are PE, PP, PVC, PET and PS, while other raw materials are destined to peculiar applications. Anyway, the most used matters are thermoplastic polymers: they can be produced and subsequently reworked with the aim of obtaining different shapes and chemical mixtures without chemical degradations.

This simple consideration highlights the role and the importance of the preventive design and end-use properties [64]. The following features can determine the initial choice of the most useful polymers:

- Resistance to tension and compression forces mechanical strength
- Heat sealability
- Optical properties (light reflection, transparency, etc.)
- Scratch resistance
- Permeability to gases and aqueous vapours.

On these bases, designers and FM may propose different containers for a single food product: the higher the number of available prototypes is, the larger will be the range of different IFP.

Moreover, the method of production can influence final properties of FP. Three different methods are recognised at present [5, 64]:

- Melting of polymers or polymer mixtures (with addition of stabilisers, colours, catalysers, etc.), extrusion and moulding (production of rigid and semirigid containers)
- Melting of polymers or polymer mixtures and realisation of thin layers by means of the passage through narrow slots or dies.

With reference to the second method, two different subprocesses may be applied [5, 64]:

- Melted mixtures are forced to pass through a narrow slot or die by means of two opposed cylinders. This 'cast' procedure is specifically used to obtain thin films and sheets for coupling or coating applications
- Melted mixtures are forced to pass through a die; subsequently, they are extruded with air pressure. This 'blow' procedure is specifically used to obtain tubular materials with specified diameters.

In addition, obtained films may be stretched in one direction (mono-oriented plastic film) or in two directions (biaxially-oriented plastic material). The aim is to strengthen mechanical resistances of films [5, 64] along one or two preferential directions: for example, the elongation may be reduced from 600 to 60 % [64]. An example of mono-oriented polymer is the linear low-density polyethylene (LLDPE); on the other side, biaxially-oriented polypropylene (BOPP) is very much appreciated for improved resistances. With reference to most used polymers, a synthetic description may be shown.

Polyethylene

PE is available in different typologies, depending on the polymeric density of produced materials. This plastic is obtained by the simple polymerisation of ethylene under high temperatures and pressures (Fig. 2.2). The density of materials is decided in the polymerisation stage [64], depending on temperatures, pressure and catalysers: in other words, polymerisation degrees may vary with the consequent decrease of 'empty spaces' in the tri-dimensional matrix of PE.

LDPE is usually considered for the production of films, sheets and other similar layered materials. It can be easily coloured (before extrusion), laminated and coupled with PP, EVA and other materials such as paperboard. LLDPE, a variety of LDPE, shows superior tensile and impact strength and puncture resistances [64].

On the opposite hand, HDPE represents the densest material. It is generally used for closures, pallets, crates, drums, rigid or semirigid containers because of the improved 'barrier effect' (impermeability to gases and water vapours) and the mechanical resistance if compared to LDPE [64]. An intermediate medium density polyethylene may be also used when HDPE properties are not strictly requested.

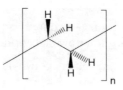

Fig. 2.2 A simplified chemical structure of polyethylene chains. BKchem version 0.13.0, 2009 (http://bkchem.zirael.org/index.html) has been used for drawing this structure

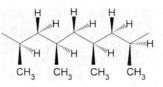
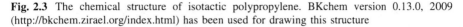

Fig. 2.3 The chemical structure of isotactic polypropylene. BKchem version 0.13.0, 2009 (http://bkchem.zirael.org/index.html) has been used for drawing this structure

Polypropylene

This polymer can be seen as the main competitor for PE in the plastic industry because of the enhanced hardness, density and transparency.

Chemically, it can be produced by propylene with a dedicated addition process by means of Ziegler-Natta type catalysers [64, 66]. The resulting chain is polymerised under pressure and heat; the structure is always ramified because of the presence of external methyl groups (Fig. 2.3). It should be considered that PP is the best available thermoplastic polymer with reference to low density, high melting point and acceptable costs if compared with other thermoplastic resins. On these bases, PP may be worked to obtain rigid and flexible FP. Moreover, this polymer may be easily coupled (extruded and laminated at the same time) with other materials, including PET, PE, EVOH and PS. The final aim is to produce high resistant temperature films for thermosealed packages: thermosealing should be carried out between 115 and 130 °C. In addition, laminated materials should at least be fit for sterilising purposes [64, 67].

Other interesting features of common PP are:

- Excellent inertness against chemical agents
- Good or acceptable barrier properties
- Low permeability to lipids
- Good resistance against plastic ageing (environmental stress cracking tests are normally very good for this material).

On the other hand, the resistance of PP to aromatic and aliphatic solvents is not good and should be ameliorated in spite of the known similarity between the above-mentioned solvents and propylene. Generally, PP can be produced also in the mono-oriented version, OPP or in the bi-dimensional type, BOPP. These materials can be easily laminated with acrylic resins with a general enhancement of all positive properties of the common PP. In addition, the problem of solvents and other impurities may be partially solved in this way [64, 68]. For these reasons, laminated acrylic/OPP and BOPP materials can substitute regenerated cellulose films.

Polystyrene

This polymer is widely known because of the versatility. In fact, the peculiarity of PS is the possible use for following products [64, 69]:

- Packed jams
- Fruit products
- Fresh meats
- Pasta
- Salads
- Cream yoghurts
- Yoghurt-based desserts
- Thermally treated milks
- Cheeses
- Margarines.

By the chemical viewpoint, PS may be seen as a different form of PP because of the substitution of methyl groups along the polymeric chain with a benzene ring (Fig. 2.4). It can be obtained by catalytic addition of styrene: the isotactic PS chain should be composed of approximately 1,000 styrene units [64, 69]. Generally, isotactic PS is known because of the adaptability to different uses; the atactic version is not good for food applications. Isotactic PS may be laminated for the production of monolayer plastic films. In addition, it can be thermoformed, moulded by injection and foamed. On these bases, isotactic PS can be used to obtain a wide range of FP.

Normal PS shows following positive features [5, 64, 69]:

- Good transparency
- High rigidity
- High chemical resistance at low temperatures;
- Good compatibility with pigments in mixtures
- Good printability
- Good thermal resistance (up to 70 °C).

On the other hand, PS films have not good barrier effects to water vapour and atmospheric gases. On these bases, PS may be suitable for the packaging of 'respiring' vegetable products. Moreover, PS is strongly attacked by aromatic solvents [69].

Another defect of common PS is the well-known fragileness. For these reasons, the biorientation and the copolymerisation with other plastic monomers—styrene

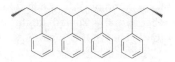

Fig. 2.4 The chemical structure of isotactic, semicrystalline polystyrene. BKchem version 0.13.0, 2009 (http://bkchem.zirael.org/index.html) has been used for drawing this structure

butadiene (SB) and acrylonitrile butadiene styrene (ABS) copolymers are well known– is recommended. The final product is known as high impact polystyrene (HIPS). Interestingly, new products can be ameliorated with the coupling with PE, PP, PET, and chemically similar polymers. Anyway, the most known form of PS is surely EPS. Fundamental properties of EPS packs are the exceptional low density and the good thermal insulation [64, 69].

Actually, nine different types at least are available at present [5]; however, only pure PS and HIPS seem to be interesting in the food sector.

Polyvinyl Chloride

By the chemical viewpoint, PVC may be seen as a different form of PP because of the substitution of methyl groups along the polymeric chain with a chloride atom (Fig. 2.5). It can be obtained by the catalytic addition of vinyl chloride. However, the normal PVC is too hard and fragile. Consequently, the addition of plasticisers is necessary; on the other hand, the original material may show interesting properties [64]. Substantially, plasticisers are needed for obtaining more workable materials: preferably, PVC without additions is used for the production of rigid trays [64]. The addition of pigments is possible and preferable [64, 69]. On the other side, PVC is cheap enough [5].

Generally, PVC is prepared in suspension and in emulsion: mass or solution procedures can be also used. Anyway, radical initiators—peroxides and azo compounds—may be needed [5]. This aspect should be carefully evaluated with relation to the migration of packaging components into foods [5, 64].

It should be also noted that PVC obtained in emulsion may absorb water; the possible aqueous absorption has to be taken into account with concern to the packaging of perishable products: moisture vapour transmission rates are notable [5, 64].

On the other hand, PVC products show low adhesiveness, good compatibility with pigments, good weldability and sticking [5]. Actually, PVC is not always used for heat- sealable packages. In fact, other PVC applications concern extruded and oriented films for wrapping [64].

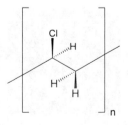

Fig. 2.5 The chemical structure of polyvinyl chloride chains. BKchem version 0.13.0, 2009 (http://bkchem.zirael.org/index.html) has been used for drawing this structure

By the chemical viewpoint, PVC is recommended for fat foods and fluids, including fruit drinks, because of the remarkable resistance to lipids. In addition, good transparency and elongation properties should be signalled, while other mechanical features—tensile strength, etc.—have to be ameliorated with plasticisers. Another big concern is the low resistance to high temperatures: the production of hydrochloric acid has to be considered; moreover, the tendency of PVC to soften when temperatures exceed 80–95 °C is well known.

Another interesting property of PVC is related to barrier effects. Actually, the permeability to aqueous vapours and other gases depends mainly on the possible addition of plasticisers: normal PVC is very good when used as a barrier for these gases; however, the higher the presence of plasticisers is, the lower will be the barrier effect [64]. For these reasons, certain PVC films for wrapping applications may be recommended for 'respiring' vegetables and 'modified atmosphere packaging' (MAP) products—red-coloured meats above all—because of the notable permeability to oxygen [64].

Finally, PCV can be produced as copolymer: polyvinylidene chloride (PVDC) is well known for the production of flexible and thermoretractable films. Chemically, vinylidene chloride and vinyl chloride monomers correspond to 80 and 20 part, respectively of the definitive copolymer. The use of PVC for heat-sealed packages is not always recommended [5, 64].

Polyesters: Polyethylene Terephthalate

Normally, food technologists and other professionals with some involvement in the food industry are accustomed to speak of 'polyesters' instead on the main polymer of this category: PET or PETE. The chemical structure of this condensation polymer is shown in Fig. 2.6.

Chemically, PET is a thermosetting polymer with melting point of 260°–265 °C. It is obtained by the condensation of terephthalic acid and ethylene glycol ester monomers. When speaking of general polyester, the condensation involves a carboxylic acid and an alcohol [5, 64]. Because of the main importance of PET in the industry of food packages, this Section is dedicated to this polymer.

PET is well known and highly recommended because of the following features [5, 64]:

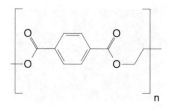

Fig. 2.6 The chemical structure of polyethylene terephthalate. BKchem version 0.13.0, 2009 (http://bkchem.zirael.org/index.html) has been used for drawing this structure

- Excellent chemical resistance to different acids
- Excellent and ameliorable resistance to vegetable oils. The copolymerisation with phenolic resins is highly recommended on condition that production costs may be affordable
- Higher heat resistance
- Remarkable mechanical strength (oriented polymers)
- Absence of shrinking below 180 °C
- Absence of processing additives for the polymerisation
- Possibility of different applications. PET can be blow- or injection-moulded, foamed, used as a coating for paperboard packages, extruded for thermo-formable and heat-sealable sheets, oriented in two directions.

For these reasons, PET is recommended for high-temperature applications, including sterilisation, 'boil in the bag', cooking or reheating packages. When used for film coating, it can be coupled with HDPE, PP, PVDC, aluminium and EVA in extruded films: obtained results are the enhancement of the initial barrier effect (discrete values for oxygen) with relation to UV light. Moreover, PET can be metallised with aluminium [5, 64]: it is a medium oxygen barrier on its own, but becomes a high barrier when coated. Another possibility for the amelioration of impermeability is the coating of PET with silica [64].

On the other hand, it should be remembered that polyesters are thermosetting polymers: they cannot be remoulded after the final hardening. In addition, the modification of mechanic resistances may be made with the variation of functional groups, while subsequent additions of peculiar chemicals may be not useful in certain situations [5].

The copolymerisation is a deal for polyesters. Thermoretractable and biodegradable co-polyesters may be obtained by means of the polycondensation with substituted amines or synthetic starch [5].

Polyamides

PA are mainly known for the important presence of the original 'nylon' brand by DuPont [64]. Chemically, PA are obtained by the condensation reaction between a diacid and a diamine. On the other hand, various possible PA can be obtained with other monomers. With reference to industrial applications for food packaging, nylon 6 and nylon 6,6 can be used as valid competitors for PET: many of excellent features of polyesters are also shown by these PA. In addition, biaxially oriented PA films demonstrate good flavour and odour barriers. Anyway, the lamination with PVDC or PE can be used to ameliorate the above-mentioned features.

On the other side, one of main problems with PA may be the excessive aqueous adsorption. This aspect is correlated with the remarkable number of peptide groups on PA chains and the increased possibility of hydrogen bonds on three molecular levels [70].

Should this adsorption exceed 2 %, mechanic resistances might be enhanced with the concomitant augment of rigidity: this phenomenon can be very important—and dangerous—when PA are moulded [5]. When speaking of MAP foods and 'respiring' vegetables, other problems may be observed [5]:

- The superficial oxidation of wetted PA films and the consequent yellow-to brown tint instead of the desired transparency
- The volumetric augment of certain packages because of the known permeability to carbon dioxide
- The strong adhesiveness, also named 'para-adhesion', between PA films and packaged foods because of the similarity between polymeric films and proteins.

Plastic Packages: Advantages and Possible Failures of the Final IFP

With relation to recognised advantages, it can be affirmed that:

- Plastic materials may be subjected to different productive processes such as moulding, extrusion, etc.
- These matters can be chemically inert and/or impermeable to different agents and food components
- Plastic polymers can be cheap enough if compared with other raw materials for similar packages
- These matters can show low density, good transparency, excellent attitudes to heat sealing and thermal processes, good or acceptable printability, etc.

These properties have been shown when discussing of PE, PP, PVC, PET and PA: in fact, the five classes of polymers can represent the whole group of plastic materials despite the presence of other extremely interesting polymers [5, 64, 69].

On the other side, possible failures of plastic FP should be discussed with relation to the safety and the integrity of the final IFP [5]. In detail, following situations should at least be considered [5]:

- Bubbling
- Undesired polymeric agglomerations—crystallites and separated accumulations—with consequent fragility and delayed fractures
- Micro fractures caused by (a) the incorrect thermal control during the orientation process and (b) heating and/or cooling steps
- Amorphous polymeric agglomerations in different zones. Causes: incorrect temperature and viscosity values during the orientation process
- Coupling failures. Examples: presence of inner creases, insufficient adhesion with air incorporation and bubbling
- Co-extrusion failures in multilayered packages. Examples: micro scratches; different flexibility of separated materials and consequent wrinkles
- Superficial opacity. Cause: reduction of extrusion-blow times with delayed and semi-amorphous polymerisation
- Moisture incorporation

- Superficial dripping, also named 'warping' or 'twisting', during the injection process
- Superficial blistering
- Other defects: flash contamination and colorimetric variations
- Partial polymerisation. When speaking of coatings for metal cans, the phenomenon is named 'partial reticulation'
- Possible transfer of chemicals from printed images
- Plastic ageing under UV exposure and excessive storage temperatures.

The discussion of the above-mentioned failures has been partially made with relation to coatings for metal can packages and glasses. Other defects have been discussed when speaking of some peculiar property of PET and PA. The interested reader is invited to consult more specific references with relation to the chemistry and the technology of packaging-related failures of food products.

2.2.8.4 Paper and Board Packages

Paper and Board (P&B) packages have a long and historical tradition in the field of food and non-food containers. The use of waxed paperboard cartons has been extensively reported in the early twentieth century and the same thing can be affirmed for the old 'paper bottle'. This coupled container, the Pure-Pack, was composed of different joint layers: paper sheets, glues, wax coatings were used as containers for cream [53, 69]. After these packages, other containers have been proposed with interesting properties. Anyway, the main feature was always the coating of paper surfaces with synthetic polymers.

From a general viewpoint, P&B packages show the following positive features [5, 53]:

- Low density
- Good stiffness
- Absence of fragileness
- Excellent printability.

In addition, P&B can be easily folded, creased and coated with adhesive products (dextrines, etc.) for the subsequent assembling.

On the other side, the following negative properties should be considered [53]:

(1) P&B materials cannot exhibit good barrier effects against water and chemical agents, including food and beverage mixtures. Paper adsorbs easily moisture, liquids and aqueous solutions
(2) At the same time, P&B packages cannot be considered good insulating containers. Actually, coating or lamination treatments may modify this property with good results
(3) Finally, paper materials do not show good tensile strength values if compared with metal supports.

On these bases, it can be affirmed that P&B packages can be used in a number of food and beverage applications. Moreover, three additional factors should be remembered [5]:

(a) Related costs are quite low if compared with other containers. P&B packages do not seem to be influenced by recurrent economic crises in the same way of other containers for non-food applications
(b) P&B packages may be reusable, recyclable, destined to the production of energy by combustion, etc.
(c) Finally, there is a virtually unlimited availability of dimensions, shapes and destinations.

At present, 50 % at least of the yearly production of P&B packages are destined to food products [5]. The following list shows several applications [71]:

• Confectionery products, including also sugar, chocolate, etc.
• Dry foods. Examples: especially bakery products, coffee, tea, etc.
• Fluid foods and other beverages
• Chilled foods
• Frozen products
• Meat, fruits and vegetables for fast consumption, with the exclusion of MAP products.

With reference to the common opinion of consumers, the main problem seems related to the identification between the so-called 'carton' and the real structure of modern P&B packages. In summary, it may be supposed that the main part of consumers consider folding cartons, paper bags and all possible P&B containers as simple accessories for foods. The superposition of different materials onto the main and structural paper support is not easily recognised.

By contrast, papers are obtained by the mixing of different raw materials [2, 5, 32, 71]:

• Vegetable fibres: cellulose, hemicellulose and lignin
• Adhesive products and glues. Examples: carboxymethylcellulose, modified resins, dextrines, etc.
• Paper colorant substances. Usually, these chemicals are inorganic pigments or optical brightness agents (OBA), also named fluorescent whitening agents
• Different additives for dry papers of synthetic origin, including PA and urea-formaldehyde resins, softeners, antistatic and antifoam chemicals
• Mineral fillers such as talc, kaolin, titanium dioxide, calcium carbonate, etc.

The use of similar formulations is strictly required for several applications. For instance, paper FP should not be formulated with the concomitant addition of glues and printing additives on the one side and mineral fillers on the other. In fact, talc or kaolin may easily reduce the superficial roughness of cellulosic plain packages with difficult printing. Moreover, the superficial hygroscopicity can be reduced.

With relation to the main support, the tripartite composition of cellulosic fibres might be questionable. However, cellulose and hemicellulose are the normal basis for cellulosic packages. On the other hand, lignin—a non-carbohydrate polymer present in wooden fibres—may be seen as a natural strengthener of wooden plants. For this and other reasons, lignin appears to be an undesired presence between cellulosic fibres [5]: excessive amounts could compromise the desired homogeneity of produced sheets.

By a general viewpoint, the difference between 'paper' and 'paperboard' packages should be also considered. Paperboard is generally thicker than paper: in addition, the last material has lower weights per square meter. In fact, ISO defines paper materials over 200 g/m^2 as 'paperboard' or 'board' sheets.

The description of the technology of production of paper materials is not the basic aim of this book. Consequently, the interested reader is invited to consult more specific literature with concern to this matter. However, the process influences basic features of P&B containers: strength, colours, thicknesses, etc. As a result, it may be synthetically explained here that paper materials can be produced by the preliminary separation between original cellulosic and non-cellulosic fibres. Actually, used raw materials can be 'virgin'—or primary—and recycled, recovered or 'secondary' sources (40–60 % of the total quantity). The chemical pulp has to be obtained by means of the effective elimination of non-cellulosic components with 'sulphate' (also known Kraft) or 'sulphite' processes [71]. Actually, recovered papers have to be de-inked; the elimination of bleaching agents in recycled papers, mineral oils, etc. has to be also carried out. After pulping, cellulosic mixtures can be sent to sheet forming procedures, but the addition of selected chemicals—water repellents such as synthetic resins, OBA, etc.—is required before this stage.

General Classification of Paper and Paperboard Types

At present, the market of commercially available P&B shows an interesting variety. Basically, the difference is related to the average length of fibres: the higher this value is, the stronger will be the resulting material. By contrast, short fibres may mean an enhanced surface smoothness [71]. This is a preliminary classification.

The origin of fibres is also important: cellulosic materials can be available as bleached, unbleached, virgin or recycled types at the same time. In addition, parameters such as grams per m^2 values and thicknesses may notably vary; the same thing may be affirmed with concern to the superficial appearance of papers and the quali-quantitative addition of chemicals [5, 71].

The following list may show many of currently appreciated solutions for the industry of P&B containers, excluding corrugated boards, boxboards, chipboards and packaging containers for secondary purposes [5, 71–74]:

- Wet strength paper. This material is resistant to water absorption. The chemical modification is obtained by the insertion of cross-linked urea formaldehyde and melamine formaldehyde. Dry polymers should correspond to a sort of paper coating. This material may be seen as a direct evolution of sack Kraft, the normal unbleached paper by sulphate treated-pulps. Grammages can vary from 70 to 100 g/m^2

- Micro creping paper. This material can be more stretched than usual
- Greaseproof, glassine and vegetable parchment types. The first material is hydrated with the aim of preventing greasy exudations (application: food products with emission of oil exudates). It can be also laminated. Glassine is a development of greaseproof papers with improved density and high glossiness. The third material is obtained by conventional chemical pulp after immersion in sulphuric acid. It shows enhanced grease resistance and wet strength
- Laminating papers (grammages: 40–80 g/m^2). These materials are both coated and uncoated papers. The composition involves pulps based on both Kraft and sulphite pulps. Subsequently, sheets can be laminated to aluminium foils and extrusion-laminated with PE
- Aluminium laminated tissues for bags, wrappings and infusible paper packages. These lightweight tissues, obtained with low chloride and sulphate traces, show notable permeability and grammages from 12 to 30 g/m^2
- Paper labels. These coated materials show grammages from 70 to 90 g/m^2
- Bag papers. These materials can be coated or uncoated, bleached or unbleached papers with 90–100 g/m^2
- Wax-coated papers. These materials are treated with fluorocarbon dispersion treatments for improving grease resistances
- Solid bleached board (SBB). This material can be easily printed, embossed, creased, cut, folded and glued. For these reasons, the design of innovative packages can easily consider the use of SBB for the preservation of aromatic foods. Chemically, the primary support is virgin paperboard obtained by bleached chemical pulp. Surfaces are coated with mineral pigments on the external side or on both sides. It is different from solid unbleached board (SUB) type because of the origin: the last paper is made from unbleached chemical pulp and colours are brown, although the coating with mineral pigments may be required. SUB may be useful when high strength and/or good wet resistances are required for liquid foods.

This list is not exhaustive, but most important types of paper materials for FP are included here. With reference to coating materials, normal solutions are LDPE, PP, LDPE/EVA, PET, PA, EVOH, and polymethylpentene and ionomer resins.

Paper and Board Containers: Advantages and Possible Failures of the Final IFP

Possible failures of P&B packages should be discussed with relation to the safety and the integrity of the final IFP [5]. In detail, many situations may be observed. Following defects should be considered at least [5], although the list could be longer:

- Increased rigidity. Substantially, the incorrect mixture of glues in the second step may generate damages and possible lacerations of obtained sheets or spools before cutting. The same failure may be also seen if excessive amounts of mineral fillers are added for whitening paper sheets. In addition, cellulosic fibres can be partially incompatible with mineral fillers. Finally, organic pigments and natural substances such as albumins may interact with fibres because of the chemical similarity
- Bleeding, also named 'ink shifting'. Main probable cause: transfer of printing inks on hydrophilic and unprinted areas in the offset printing technique
- Flexographic defects. Examples: incorrect drying, residual absorption of water or organic molecules with the consequent softening of printed materials
- Chromatic variations. Causes: presence of natural substances such as albumins with the consequent yellow tint under light exposure; excessive amount of OBA
- Wrinkling. Cause: initial pulp mixtures do not appear homogeneous. Cellulosic fibres are not amalgamated as expected because of the incorrect viscosity
- Other failures: defective adhesion, pulverisation of supports. Cause: excessive moisturisation of paper supports and raw materials during the storage in humid warehouses
- Mildewing by moulds (microbial spreading). Cause: storage in contaminated and humid warehouses.

References

1. Pastore A, Vernuccio M (2004) Il packaging nel processo di consumo: prospettive di analisi tra Semiotica e Marketing. Finanz Mark Prod 3:108–137. ISSN:1593-2230
2. Piergiovanni L, Limbo S (2010) Materiali, Tecnologie E Qualità Degli Alimenti. Springer-Verlag Italia, Milan
3. Hartman Group: Ideas in Food (2013) A cultural perspective. The Hartman Group, Inc. http://www.hartman-group.com/downloads/white-papers/ideas-in-food-2013. Accessed 14 Dec 2013
4. Lasserre P (2007) Globalization of mass retail. In: Macmillan P (ed) Global Strategic Management Mini Cases Series. http://www.philippelasserre.net/contenu/Download/Mass_Retail.pdf. Accessed 27 Jan 2014
5. Parisi S (2012) Food packaging and food alterations: the user-oriented approach. Smithers Rapra Technology, Shawbury
6. Bucchetti V (2005) Packaging design. Storia, linguaggi, progetto. Franco Angeli, Milan
7. Brunazzi G (2009) Hello! Logos. Logos, Modena
8. Brunazzi G (ed) (1997) Dizionario del package design (A to Z of package design terminology). Burgo, Torino
9. Bhalla V, Grimm PC, Chertow GM, Pao AC (2009) Melamine nephrotoxicity: an emerging epidemic in an era of globalization. Kidney Int 75(8):774–779. doi:10.1038/ki.2009.16
10. Parisi S (2013) Food industry and packaging materials—performance-oriented guidelines for users. Smithers Rapra Technology, Shawbury
11. Rundh B (2005) The multi-faceted dimension of packaging: Marketing logistic or marketing tool? Br Food J 107(9):670–684. doi:10.1108/00070700510615053

12. Sacharow S (2006) Shelf life extension using packaging techniques. In: Havkin-Frenkel D, Frenkel C, Dudai N (eds) First international symposium on natural preservatives in food systems, Princeton, 2005. Acta Horticulturae, No 709, vol 1. International Society for Horticultural Science, Leuven
13. Cagnon T, Méry A, Chalier P, Guillaume C, Gontard N (2013) Fresh food packaging design: a requirement driven approach applied to strawberries and agro-based materials. Innovat Food Sci Emerg Tech 20:288–298. doi:10.1016/j.ifset.2013.05.009
14. Pereno A (2012) Tra comunicazione e prodotto: il packaging. In: Tamborrini P, Barbero S (eds) Il Fare Ecologico. Il prodotto industriale e i suoi requisiti ambientali. Edizione Ambiente, Milan, pp 88–90
15. Marsh K, Bugusu B (2007) Food packaging—roles, materials, and environmental issues. J Food Sci 72(3):39–55. doi:10.1111/j.1750-3841.2007.00301.x
16. Ottaviani F (2002) Il metodo HACCP (Hazard analysis and critical control points). In: Andreis G, Ottaviani F (eds) Manuale di sicurezza degli alimenti. Principi di ecologia microbica e di legislazione applicati alla produzione alimentare. Oxoid S.p.A., G. Milanese
17. Micali M, Parisi S, Minutoli E, Delia S, Laganà P (2009) Alimenti confezionati e atmosfera modificata. Caratteristiche basilari, nuove procedure, applicazioni pratiche. Ind Aliment 489:35–43
18. Privat K, Thonart P (2011) Protective action of cultures: The case of lactic bacteria against undesirable food flora. Biotechnol Agron Soc Environ 15(2):339–348. ISSN:1370-6233
19. Parisi S, Delia S, Laganà P (2008a) Typical Italian cheeses and polymeric coatings. Recommended guidelines for food companies. Parts I and II. Food Package Bull 17(7&8):17–21
20. Parisi S, Delia S, Laganà P (2008b) Typical Italian Cheeses and Polymeric Coatings. Recommended Guidelines For Food Companies. Parts III. Food Packag Bull 17, 10:12-15
21. Parisi S (2009) Intelligent Packaging for the Food Industry. In: Carter EJ (ed) Polymer electronics—a flexible technology. Smithers Rapra Technology Ltd, Shawbury
22. Inns GR (2012) The packaging supply chain. In: Emblem A, Emblem H (eds) Packaging technology: fundamentals, materials and processes. Woodhead Publishing Limited, Cambridge, pp 10–23
23. Bastian J, Zentes J (2013) Supply chain transparency as a key prerequisite for sustainable agri-food supply chain management. Int Rev Retail Distrib Consum Res 23(5):553–570. doi:10.1080/09593969.2013.834836
24. Pezzoli P (2012) Resealable packaging container with interior mounted pressure sensitive coated collar. US Patent 2,014,000,021, 29 giu 2012
25. Margolin V (2013) Design studies and food studies: parallels and intersections. Des Cult 5(3):375–392. doi:10.2752/175470813X13705953612327
26. Italian Institute of Packaging (2013) Linee guida per la valutazione dell'idoneità al contatto con alimenti del packaging realizzato con materiale proveniente da riciclo. The Italian Institute of Packaging, Milan
27. Kernoghan N (2012) Mineral oil in recycled paper and board packaging. Smithers Pira. https://www.smitherspira.com/testing/food-contact/ news-free-webinar-mineral-oil-in-recycled-paper-and-board-packaging.aspx. Accessed 11 Oct 2013
28. Vollmer A, Biedermann M, Grundböck F, Ingenhoff J-E, Biedermann-Brem S, Altkofer W, Grob K (2011) Migration of mineral oil from printed paperboard into dry foods: survey of the German market. Eur Food Res Technol 232:175–182. doi:10.1007/s00217-010-1376-6
29. Eurostat (2013) Packaging waste statistics. http://epp.eurostat.ec.europa.eu/statistics_ explained/index.php/Packaging_waste_statistics. Accessed 17 Dec 2013
30. Wiedmann T, Minx J (2008) A definition of 'carbon footprint'. In: Pertsova CC (ed) Ecological economics research trends: chapter 1. Nova Science Publishers, Hauppauge, pp 1–11
31. Ashby M, Johnson K (2010) Materials and design: the art and science of material selection in product design, 2nd edn. Elsevier, Philadelphia

32. Ottenio D, Escabasse JY, Podd B (2004) Packaging materials 6. Paper and board for food packaging applications. ILSI Europe Rep Ser 2004:1–24
33. Barbero S, Pereno A, Tamborrini P (2011) Qualitative/quantitative cross analysis to design eco-pack. In: Castillo L, Guedes M, Franklin W (eds) Proceedings of the 3rd international symposium on sustainable design (III ISSD), Recife, Sept 2011. Editora Universitària UFPE, pp 105–115
34. Shinkman M, Lewis P (2008) Rich pickings, opportunities in South-east Asia's emerging markets. Atradius Credit Insurance NV and The Economist Intelligence Unit, Westbury, p.15. http://www.asia-now.com/files/ideas/Rich%20pickings%20Opportunities%20in%20South %20East%20Asia's%20emerging%20markets.pdf. Accessed 28 Jan 2014
35. Ciravegna E (2010) La qualità del packaging. Franco Angeli, Milano
36. Parisi S (2004) Alterazioni in imballaggi metallici termicamente processati. Gulotta Press, Palermo
37. Bucchetti V (2001) PackAge: storia, costume, industria, funzioni e futuro dell'imballaggio. Lupetti, Milan
38. Olins W (1989) Corporate identity. Thames and Hudson, London
39. Brunazzi G (1993) Corporate Identity 3. Package design. Ghiorzo Editore, Milan
40. MacRae R, Szabo M, Anderson K, Louden F, Trillo S (2012) Empowering the citizen-consumer: re-regulating consumer information to support the transition to sustainable and health promoting food systems in Canada. Sustainability 4(9):2146–2175. doi:10.3390/su4092146
41. De Nardo LM (2009) Food packaging: designing with the consumer. Elledì, Milan
42. Pereno A, Tamborrini P (2013) Packaging as a means for promoting sustainable and aware consumption. In: Proceedings of 4th international symposium on sustainable design, Federal University of Rio Grande do Sul, Porto Alegre, 12–14 Nov 2013
43. Lowe B, de Souza-Monteiro DM, Fraser I (2013) Nutritional labelling information: utilisation of new technologies. J Mark Manag 29(11–12):1337–1366. doi:10.1080/0267257X.2013. 798673
44. Barbero S, Cozzo B (2009) Ecodesign. H.F. Ullmann, Königswinter
45. Sutter J, Dudler V, Meuwly R (2011) Packaging materials 8. Printing inks for food packaging composition and properties of printing inks. ILSI Europe Ser 2011:1–32
46. Tamborrini P (2009) Design sostenibile. Oggetti, sistemi e comportamenti. Electa, Milan
47. Grönman K, Soukka R, Järvi-Kääriäinen T, Katajajuuri JM, Kuisma M, Koivupuro HK, Ollila M, Pitkänen M, Miettinen O, Silvenius F, Thun R, Wessman H, Linnanen L (2013) Framework for Sustainable Food Packaging Design. Package Technol Sci 26(4):187–200. doi:10.1002/pts.1971
48. Germak C (2008) Man at the centre of the project. Allemandi, Torino
49. Hanss D, Böhm G (2012) Sustainability seen from the perspective of consumers. Int J Consum Stud 36(6):678–687. doi:10.1111/j.1470-6431.2011.01045.x
50. Bennett JW, Bentley R (2000) Seeing red: the story of prodigiosin. Adv Appl Microbiol 47:1–32. doi:10.1016/S0065-2164(00)47000-0
51. Parisi S (2002) Profili evolutivi dei contenuti batterici e chimico-fisici in prodotti lattiero-caseari. Ind Aliment 412:295–306
52. Parisi S (2003) Evoluzione chimico-fisica e microbiologica nella conservazione di prodotti lattiero - caseari. Ind Aliment 423:249–259
53. Coles R (2003) Introduction. In: Coles R, McDowell D, Kirwan MJ (eds) Food packaging technology. Blackwell Publishing Ltd, Oxford
54. Page B, Edwards M, May N (2003) Metal cans. In: Coles R, McDowell D, Kirwan MJ (eds) Food packaging technology. Blackwell Publishing Ltd, Oxford
55. Pilley KP (1981) Lacquers, varnishes and coatings for food and drink cans and for the decorating industry. Arthur Holden Surface Coatings Ltd, Birmingham
56. Girling PJ (2003) Packaging of food in glass containers. In: Coles R, McDowell D, Kirwan MJ (eds) Food packaging technology. Blackwell Publishing Ltd, Oxford

57. Falcone R (2012) Raw materials and glass analyses. http://www.glasstrend.nl/uploads/files/
    Microsoft%20PowerPoint%20-%205b%20SSV%20Raw%20Materials%20&%20Glass%20
    Analyses.pdf. Accessed 29 Apr 2014
58. Wang C, Tao Y (2003) The weathering of silicate glasses. J Chin Ceram Soc 31(1):78–85
59. Walters HV, Adams PB (1975) Effects of humidity on the weathering of glass. J Non-Cryst
    Solids 19:183–199. doi:10.1016/0022-3093(75)90084-8
60. Snyder HM (1990) Cold-end coatings in glass container manufacture. Am Ceram Soc Bull
    69(11):1831–1833
61. Gierenz G, Karmann W (eds) (2008) Adhesives and adhesive tapes. Wiley-VCH Verlag
    GmbH, Weinheim
62. Wang LD, Du FG, Shi JP (2006) Water-resistant paper-label adhesive for high-speed
    labeling. Adhes China 4:001
63. Pérez-Coello MS, Díaz-Maroto MC (2009) Volatile compounds and wine aging. In: Moreno-
    Arribas MV, Polo MC (eds) Wine chemistry and biochemistry. Springer, New York,
    pp 295–311. doi:10.1007/978-0-387-74118-5_16
64. Monagas M., Bartolomé B, Gómez-Cordovés C (2005) Evolution of polyphenols in red wines
    from Vitis vinifera L. during aging in the bottle. Eur Food Res Technol 220(3–4):331–340.
    doi:10.1016/j.foodchem.2005.01.004
65. Kirwan MJ, Strawbridge JW (2003) Plastics in food packaging. In: Coles R, McDowell D,
    Kirwan MJ (eds) Food packaging technology. Blackwell Publishing Ltd, Oxford
66. Castonguay LA, Rappe AK (1992) Ziegler-Natta catalysis. A theoretical study of the isotactic
    polymerization of propylene. J Amer Chem Soc 114(14):5832–5842. doi:10.1021/ja00040a053
67. Johnston WD (1987). Laminate film for flexible containers. US Patent 4,654,240, 31 Mar
    1987
68. Song YS, Begley T, Paquette K, Komolprasert V (2003) Effectiveness of polypropylene film
    as a barrier to migration from recycled paperboard packaging to fatty and high-moisture food.
    Food Add Contam 20(9):875–883. doi:10.1080/02652030310001597592
69. Robertson GL (2002) The paper beverage carton: past and future. Food Technol 56(7):46–52
70. Parisi S, Laganà P, Stilo A, Micali M, Piccione D, Delia S (2009) Il massimo assorbimento
    idrico nei formaggi. Tripartizione del contenuto acquoso per mole d'azoto. Ind Aliment
    491:31–41
71. Kirwan MJ (2003) Paper and paperboard packaging. In: Coles R, McDowell D, Kirwan MJ
    (eds) Food packaging technology. Blackwell Publishing Ltd, Oxford
72. Kirwan MJ (2012) Paper-based flexible packaging. In: Handbook of Paper and Paperboard
    Packaging Technology, 2nd edn. Wiley, Oxford. doi: 10.1002/9781118470930.ch3
73. Brody AL (1997) Packaging, food. In: Brody AL, Marsh KS (eds) The wiley encyclopedia of
    packaging technology, 2nd edn. Wiley, New York, pp 699–704
74. Jarnberg T, Landqvist N, Nordin B, Spangenberg S (1988) Manufacturing of kraft paper. US
    Patent 4,741,376, 3 May 1988

Chapter 3
The Instrumental Role of Food Packaging

Abstract Packaging are physical 'media' which aim to satisfy three main requirements: to contain, preserve and transport human products. Functionality is the real essence of the synergetic food/packaging system. However, there is not functionality without communication. The concept of food packaging concerns a dualistic system: on the one side, every food packaging is expected to preserve packaged foods against thermal leaps, environmental moisture, mechanical damages (functional requirements). The viewpoint of research chemists is important: all above mentioned factors depend also on chemical processes, analytical methods, food examinations and reports when speaking of human health, food safety, logistic matters and environmental sustainability of recycling processes. On the other hand, packaging design enhances the communication. Consequently, the complex relationship between communication (according to a design approach) and functional requirements has to be carefully studied in the pre-production step.

Keywords Food packaging material · Integrated food product · Active packaging · Intelligent packaging · Remaining shelf life · Food protection · Food preservation · Logistics · Disposal · Usage requirements · Visual communication

Abbreviations

Biaxially oriented polypropylene	BOPP
European Union	EU
Ethylene acrylic acid	EAA
Food manufacturer	FM
Food packaging	FP
Food packaging producer	FPP
Hazard analysis and critical control points	HACCP
Information technology	IT
In-mould shield	IMS
Integrated food product	IFP
Intelligent packaging	IP
International featured standard	IFS
Low density polyethylene	LDPE

© The Author(s) 2014
G. Brunazzi et al., *The Importance of Packaging Design for the Chemistry of Food Products*, SpringerBriefs in Chemistry of Foods,
DOI: 10.1007/978-3-319-08452-7_3

57

Modified atmosphere packaging   MAP
Normal temperature indicator   NTI
Packaging machinery system   FPS
Polypropylene   PP
Radio frequency identification   RFID
Remaining shelf life   RSL
Shelf ready packaging   SRP
Technological suitability   TS
Time-temperature indicator   TTI
Ultraviolet   UV
Vertical form-fill   VFF

3.1 Introduction

Packages are first of all physical 'media' which aim to satisfy three main requirements: to contain, preserve and transport human products. This simplified and essential description can be considered still valid today for food packaging (FP) in spite of evident or 'transparent' superstructures [1].

Substantially, it can be affirmed that the functional aspect of FP is the real essence of the simplified and synergetic food/packaging system, also defined the 'integrated food product' (Sect. 1.1). Actually, there is not functionality without communication. As a result, it should be honestly considered that the whole system of requirements and features of a modern FP is dependent on functional (mechanical, technological, chemical, microbiological, sensorial) factors of the 'integrated food product' (IFP) and communicative strategies of FP at the same time. In other words, the conceptual idea of FP has to be seen as a dualistic system.

However, the first and tangible nature of packaging is surely dependent from functional requirements: this obligation is extremely evident when speaking of FP because of the main 'weight' of practical features in comparison with other indefinite needs [2, 3].

First of all, every FP has to preserve its own content after the final packaging step and until a specified temporal limit (Sect. 1.1). Secondly, the delivery of packaged foods has to be allowed and possibly simplified; at the same time, storage requirements have to be easily satisfied. Moreover, the use of final IFP should be actively promoted by means of peculiar FP features; finally, the management of wastes should be taken into account. By a simplistic viewpoint, this list should be exhaustive; however, every IFP has different needs depending on the particular food category [4]. So, the higher the diversification of IFP on the market, the higher the correlated diversification of FP.

Generally, the first relationship between the packaging and the packaged food corresponds to the dimensional property: this aspect is strongly dependent on the chemistry of materials and finished food products. In spite of this obvious concept, the current situation of available FP on the market appear redundant from the functional viewpoint. The following list of unsatisfactory performances may be helpful:

- Excessive protection against crashes
- Excessive dimensions and/or thickness
- Insufficient ergonomic features of the final IFP
- Difficult opening.

As a result, FP may be fit for the intended use: this concept is part of the definition of 'technological suitability' (TS) of food contact approved materials in the European Union (EU) according to Parisi [5]. By contrast, several FP cannot comply with required or tacitly communicated features of packaged foods because of their excessive or deficient properties.

The impact of this situation on different matters should be taken into account, including environmental sustainability and marketing strategies also: low functionality can surely influence the perceived value of the final IFP with obvious negative results.

On the other side, the importance of the initial FP design has to be highlighted. Normally, the cooperation between the food packaging producer (FPP), the food manufacturer (FM) and the supplier of packaging machinery systems (FPS) is highly desirable. As a clear consequence, the realisation—and the desirable success—of the first FP prototype may depend on following factors:

- The careful selection of raw materials for FP
- The selection of most useful technologies for FP manufacturing
- The 'right' decision of analytical procedures with reference to

  - The reliable definition of TS for FP against the final IFP, and
  - Requirements of the whole distribution chain.

Clearly, the viewpoint of research chemists is important: all above mentioned factors depend strongly on chemical processes, analytical methods, food examinations and reports when speaking of human health, food safety and environmental sustainability of recycling processes. For these reasons, this book shows different case studies in which the problem of design is analysed in two ways:

- The viewpoint of designers (they have to comply with different marketing requirements and users' needs)
- The opinion of research chemists with different specialisations and competencies.

With concern to the first point, designers have to take into account users' needs before analysing other important requirements; cultural codes may restrict IFP uses depending on the original target [6].

At the same time, receivers of marketing strategies—category of consumers, organisations, ethical communities, etc.—may influence the choice of functional features: ergonomic features, shape, weights, materials, opening and closure devices, self-heating or self-cooling inner systems, performances of IFP along different steps of the food chain. All these features of the complex relationship between communication and functional requirements have to be considered in the design step. Otherwise, the commercial success of IFP cannot be reliably predicted or other 'grotesque' situations can occur.

For example, the competition between different but similar packaging can favour one only of these FP when all competitors are designed and 'built' with one single and widely recognised archetype [7, 8].

3.2 Foods and Functions

Packaging and packaged products are interconnected: the result may be defined 'integrated food/packaging system'. Certainly, the synergic interconnection becomes more complex if the packaged good is edible. From the viewpoint of technologists and material scientists, two factors have to be considered because of their 'mandatory' (stringent) meaning: the perishability and the edibility. The first of these two features is strictly linked to the problem of the 'remaining shelf life' (RSL) assessment. RSL values can be remarkable (extended durability) or very low (rapid perishability): anyway, their assessment depends on evolving profiles of different parameters [9]:

- Microbial counts, with concern to degrading micro organisms and pathogenic agents
- Undesirable chemical analytes (examples: sulphur amino acids, enzymatic browning and Maillard reaction- products, histamine in fish products, etc.)
- Organoleptic performances (taste, colour, smell, shape, texture).

On the other side, the edibility is connected with regulatory requirements and other factors concerning food and non-food materials and processes. One of these aspects is surely the positive or negative influence of FP: food containers have to preserve edible products without unacceptable alterations [2]. In other terms in large-scale retail trade, every packaged food needs to be improved and enhanced in comparison with the original and unpackaged edible good. As a consequence, industrial IFP can be considered the 'updated' version of the original food with enhanced appearance; in addition, 'empowered' food features (chemical features, sensorial aspect, etc.) would be requested to remain constant during long temporal periods.

On these bases, three main categories of FP features may be discussed:

1. Reactivity of IFP to environmental moisture and thermal leaps
2. Protection against crashes
3. Safety and hygiene.

Every IFP is constantly subjected to notable variations during the whole extension of the 'food chain'. FP are specifically expected to preserve packaged foods against thermal leaps and environmental moisture when foods are defined 'easily perishable' (notable variations in very restricted times) or 'perishable'.

At the same time, packaged foods can suffer mechanical damages because of sudden bumps in spite of the mechanic nature of suffered defects (ruptures of FP, etc.). Real consequences are often: microbial spreading; organoleptic modifications, colorimetric variations above all; oxidative reactions (target molecules: fatty acids, etc.); and other failures.

Finally, FP have to be 'hygiene and safety'-compliant: from a general viewpoint, this affirmation should be related at least to the absence of microbial contamination and harmful or toxic chemical analytes. Moreover, the 'Hazard Analysis and Critical Control Points' (HACCP) approach considers these dangers and other possibilities. One of the most discussed concerns appears linked to nanomaterials in FP; another big matter is often linked (Sect. 2.2.4) to chemical contaminants from recycling processes. In particular, this debate is 'thorny' enough because of the apparent role of secondary packaging (Sect. 2.2.2) in spite of the complete absence of food contact interactions [10, 11].

Finally, the role of different food macro-categories [12] should be highlighted because of the profound influence on the modification of FP functions. Several case studies—common FP and related IFP—are shown in this book with the aim of discussing positive connections between main food typologies and consequent FP features [13].

3.3 Protection and Preservation Requirements

Main functional features of FP—preservation and protection (Sect. 2.2.1)—are generally dependent on the particular food macro-category, while the interaction with human manufacturers, distributors and customers can have little influence. Anyway, preservation and protection are similar and often confused concepts because of their strong interconnection. As a result, the choice of a peculiar design depends on the consideration of both functions.

As mentioned in Sect. 2.2.1, protection concerns the defence of the packaged product and the whole IFP by external attacks: powders, ultraviolet (UV) rays, thermal leaps, moisture, crashes, compression, vibrations, etc. On the opposite side, preservation concerns the protection against microbiological agents: degrading micro organisms (yeasts, moulds, etc.), pathogenic bacteria, correlated degrading chemical reactions [2, 14].

By the chemical viewpoint, FP design should comply with different requirements: the protection of inner gases (oxygen above all) and moisture (the inner atmosphere is constantly in contact with food surfaces); the preservation against environmental moisture, heating, UV or infrared radiations.

In detail, it should be clarified that the protection of the IFP against chemical agents is effectively obtained by means of suitable materials (low permeability from the external side, good permeability outside the inner product; excellent mechanical resistance against breakages and damages, etc.) and closure systems. Furthermore, the coupling of materials with different chemical nature may be very useful when food products are preserved with the 'modified atmosphere packaging' (MAP) technology [5, 15].

Moreover, mechanical performances of packaged products are preserved if FP can resist to bumps, abrasions, vibrations, etc.

So the choice of FP materials is critical and dependent on chemical features and mechanical performances. Obviously, these factors have to be constantly evaluated and revalidated (example: infrangibility of certain glass jars) according to recognised analytical protocols or validated methods by the FM and the FPP: the joint validation should be always welcomed [5].

Certainly, the correct design of FP shapes is useful for assuring good physical protection to IFP: known examples concern the correct placement and stability of packaged goods into the container in all possible transport conditions. On the other side, new or innovative shapes can be designed and proposed with the aim of helping the future destination of FP as waste [16, 17].

The microbiological problem cannot be excluded when speaking of FP, in spite of the clear and undeniable origin of employed materials. The protection of IFP is mainly connected to inner FP conditions: foods may be easily perishable when pathogen agents and degrading micro organisms can spread without opposition. In addition, external microbiological contaminations have to be avoided: generally, following mechanisms are responsible for food perishability:

- Attack by environmentally diffused life forms
- Contamination by microbial aggregates on FP surfaces (despite the non-edible nature of packaging)
- Attack by insects and/or rodents
- Transmission of peculiar odours (these gaseous emissions may be defined microbiological 'carriers' because of aerosolised dispersions)
- Transmission of aerosolised suspensions on inner FP surfaces (before packaging operations) and subsequent adherence on food surfaces.

The last of these mechanisms is also defined FP 'passive microbial contamination' [5, 18]. Anyway, the answer to these contamination dangers is linked to the correct design of FP (choice of good materials; fit closure systems). Additionally, every possible microbial spreading (and related consequences on IFP) is also dependent on unfit or incorrect storage conditions without FP damages. In other words, closed and undamaged FP might cause microbiological failures when incorrect storage conditions are demonstrated; should this situation occur, food analysts could conclude that the 'perfection' of used FP—good closure, excellent waterproofing, etc.—may determine the decrease of the remaining shelf life (RSL) when the IFP is badly stored [5, 19].

Anyway, FP have to be carefully designed because of two specific purposes (Sect. 1.1):

(a) To maintain the qualitative and quantitative level of the original IFP where possible
(b) To increase RSL values.

These requirements can be satisfied by means of new FP: currently, 'old' packages are usually proposed with several innovative developments. On the other side, new concepts have been proposed with notable results and good future perspectives: 'smart' packages, also named 'active' packaging (because of the declared interaction with the food). In addition, 'intelligent' packaging systems [20] have other important functions (easy RSL or temperature monitoring and/or recording).

Generally, active packaging is well considered in the market of FP because of the constant and 'active' interaction with edible surfaces. This objective can be obtained by means of the extension of expected RSL values in comparison with the original (natural, unpackaged) food product [20]. Colorimetric variations become significantly slower than expected, textural modifications of the inner food and the whole IFP are less evident during the time, normal chemical reactions at the food/atmosphere interface are kinetically less favoured. For example, the well known 'respiration' phenomenon into 'ready-to-eat' packaged vegetables is notably inhibited by the synergic action of MAP systems and active release packaging devices [15]. Consequently, RSL values of MAP vegetables can be enhanced in comparison with unpackaged foods with the concomitant use of active devices.

However, there are several conceptual differences in the whole class of 'smart' or 'active packages'. Indeed, the general term 'active packaging' is referred to two different typologies of interactive devices. The main difference concerns the capacity of interaction with foods [20].

Normal 'active packaging' systems are defined in this specific way because of their active interaction with inner atmospheres and packaged foods: naturally, this interaction has to be correctly interpreted by food technologists in terms of important modifications of packaged products and related atmospheres by means of antimicrobial and/or antioxidant substances [20]. Several of these solutions can absorb external substances (for example: oxygen) while other systems are able to release useful gases (example: ethylene, for packaged fruits). By this viewpoint, one or more sensorial features of packaged products are visibly and undoubtedly altered: colour, smell, texture, perceived shape, etc. Consequently, RSL values have to be re-evaluated because of the influence of organoleptic properties on durability and microbial ecologies [18, 20]. Other active packaging can limit or prevent the microbial spreading by means of the release of natural or synthetic substances into the inner FP atmosphere [2, 15, 21].

On the other hand, smart packaging systems can be subdivided in two categories depending on used technologies. The first subclass is related to connectable hardware and software products: Radio Frequency Identification (RFID) devices.

Currently, RFID tags may have serious difficulties because of high costs for the complete implementation of related computer systems [20]. It may be assumed that new 'multifactor tags' (a combination of chemicals, inks and coatings with RFID) may reduce real costs [20]. Anyway, the most important advantage—distances between the main software centre system and RFID tags can reach 30 m—should be considered with the true reason for high costs: every tag was evaluated $100 before 2010 [20].

It may be useful to know that RFID systems are a three-component application into very small areas (generally, one square centimetre only). Three elements are needed for the realisation of useful RFID adhesive tags [20]:

- A dedicated transponder
- An identification code (it represents thousands of bits of unwritten but potential information)
- Low batteries or solar micro-cells
- The mini-antenna.

The aim of this three-level composition is to allow the transmission and the reception of predetermined signals by means of transponders [20]. This description may be really complicated for inexperienced readers. On the other hand, such a design cannot affect basic IFP appearances because of their dimensions: RFID tags may be adhesive labels, bottoms or micro-ampoules [20].

The second 'intelligent' category concerns all specifically designed systems for the collection, storage and visual interpretation of historical information and physicochemical information about the whole IFP [18, 20]. Usually, these systems are connected internally or externally to used FP. In detail, related functions may be described as follows [18, 22]:

- Detection of storage conditions versus time: targeted parameters are temperature and relative humidity above all
- Demonstration of qualitative or quantitative failures, defects or variations into IFP after a specified temporal period
- Detection of storage conditions and qualitative or quantitative failures, failings or variations at the same time.

The final action of smart packaging systems is always the reliable storage of above mentioned relevant information. More specifically, the following classification may be shown and synthetically discussed.

Currently, active packaging systems are based on RFID technology: IFP can be easily monitored during transportation and storage steps and during all the shelf life. Storage temperatures are extremely interesting values in the food industry because of possible health and safety controls and the existing risk of 'class-action' procedures by consumer associations [18, 20]. Moreover, relative humidity may interest food technologists; the same thing can be assumed with reference to partial pressure values of oxygen (perishable foods).

In relation to intelligent packaging (IP) systems, the most part of food complaints is strictly related to storage conditions and RSL. For these reasons, IP are normally classified as follows [18, 22, 23]:

- Normal temperature indicators (NTI) and time-temperature indicators (TTI)
- Leakage indicators
- Freshness indicators.

Generally, NTI and TTI are often confused [18] in spite of profound differences between these systems. In fact, NTI are simple thermal recorders and the collected information is substantially irreversible because the maximum temperature is displayed without other information. On the other side, TTI can easily display collected thermal values versus time. Visual results may be considered the average sum of all thermal variations. Visible modifications concern RSL: This parameter is displayed in a colorimetric way and chromatic variations are generally associated to IFP quality.

Moreover, current TTI solutions—chromatographic solutions, 'bull's eye' systems, enzymatic indicators—can be easily 'read' and interpreted by food technologists and common consumers [18].

Leakage and freshness indicators should be also mentioned. Leakage systems can detect undesired oxygen and/or carbon dioxide into MAP packages by means of redox indicators or acid/base systems. On the other side, freshness indicators are specifically designed for detecting gaseous substances by microbial spoilage: ammonia, tri-methylamine N-oxide, hydrogen sulphide, etc. [18]. Differently from TTI and NTI, common consumers may recognise these systems as extraneous or incompatible with fresh foods. This situation should be carefully considered by FM.

3.4 Transport and Storage Requirements

Packaging must comply with different needs, including transportation and storage requirements. These can be defined as 'traditional' needs because packaging has always been a device to transport and handle products. Consequently, every food or non-food packaging is primarily designed to comply with these needs. With concern to edible products, FP are surely requested to make easier delivery and storage operations; furthermore, unpackaged foods can be liquid, solid, powdered and/or deformable and IFP may be poorly ergonomic. Thus, good or reliable FP—and resulting IFP—should easily allow the management of transportation, warehousing and storage operations on a large (national or international) scale.

Within industrial transportation and storage operations, the basic unit is normally the association of three different typologies of packaging:

- The primary packaging: i.e. the basic IFP unit of sale, with a dedicated lot number

- The secondary packaging: it contains 'n' equal IFP. A peculiar barcode may be associated with every secondary package where possible (and accepted by FP)
- The tertiary packaging: it collects 'm' secondary packaging into a third level-packaging with a simplified structure (wooden pallet; plastic wrapping films or large bags); optional paper or metal dividers and a dedicated barcode, where possible (and accepted by FP).

The correct design of IFP, secondary packages and the final assembling of the tertiary packaging, has the aim of reducing 'empty spaces' into containers and cargos [24], with concomitant cost reductions. In fact, following 'voices' should be considered before studying the best FP:

- Environmental sustainability of transportation
- Energy consumption, also named 'carbon footprint' (Sect. 2.2.2)
- Use of recycled materials
- Logistic costs.

With reference to the last factor, logistics concerns:

- Number of necessary travels
- Booking of intermediate warehouses, where necessary
- Transport costs.

On these bases, new solutions have been recently proposed. One of the last examples is the 'Shelf Ready Packaging' (SRP): this secondary container is designed to be opened, placed on shelves and used as a display for IFP. The first and original function of the secondary packaging—the easy warehousing—has been substantially modified if compared with classic cardboard boxes. Indeed, the SRP allows the reduction of packaging-related costs and processes. An interesting case study may be considered with reference to packaged chips and similar food products. Normally, this typology of fried foods is packed into laminated and flexible packages with different shapes and dimensions.

Different approaches may be suggested for the above mentioned case study. Probably, the best strategy should be multidisciplinary and correlated to the specificity of the packaged product. For this reason, the discussion will concern initially the food product. Subsequently, two food packaging applications will be displayed with possible risks and advantages.

3.4.1 Food Product: Fried Potato Chips in Thermosealed Pouches

Fried potato chips belong to the general category of snack foods. By a general viewpoint, the peculiarity of these products is surely the subdivision of a relatively small amount of edible foods in a number of pieces. For example, 100 gms of chips may be offered as the correspondent quantity of 1.5 gms—pieces; however, the number of individual slices is 67 at least. Consequently, every possible physicochemical reaction and subsequent degradations are extremely enhanced with comparison with the undivided food because of the enormous augment of superficial areas [25].

With relation to the increase of superficial areas, the main problem for fried potato chips appears linked to rancidity [26]. In other words, the secondary oxidation of used oils for frying processes may cause the progressive accumulation of malondialdehyde and other chemical substances during storage. This variation is shown by the development of rancid odours and off-flavours [27]. In addition, it should be considered that the oxidation speed of saturated fatty acids is notably lower if compared with unsaturated fatty acids [26]. Generally, the oxidation of fatty acids is initiated in the deep-fat frying process by the formation of free radicals in presence of metal ions, heating or light exposure (Fig. 3.1).

With exclusive reference to fried potato chips, a remarkable correlation has been shown between the reduction of oxidation and the extension of barrier effects in packaging films [26]. In detail, it has been reported that the effect of light exposure and environmental moisture may reduce the shelf life of packaged products because of rancid odours; on the other side, it appears that textural modifications by moisture adsorption are less important [26].

With reference to this case study, normal fried potato chips can be considered for an industrial process. Fried chips have been obtained by fresh potatoes after peeling and automatic slicing. The final thickness of chips should be approximately between 2 and 3 mm. Subsequently, sliced chips may be subjected to the so-called deep-fat frying process (approximate temperature: 180 °C) with the use of vegetable oils such as cottonseed, sunflower and safflower oils or hydrogenated vegetable oils [28].

The qualitative evaluation can be made by different methods. With reference to rancidity, the analysis of peroxide values, iodine value, free fatty acid content, fatty acid composition, the composition of carbonylic compounds such as p-anisidine value, and the evaluation of UV absorbance at 232 and 268 nm can be recommended [27, 29, 30]. A modest augment in the weight of fried pieces might be observed because of the addition of oxygen to lipids and the consequent formation of hydroperoxides during the initial auto-oxidation.

3.4.2 Fried Potato Chips in Thermosealed Pouches: Possible Packaging Solutions

Different solutions may be available with relation to the packaging of fried chips and similar snack foods: for example, multilayered rigid tubular containers made by polypropylene, aluminium foil, polyethylene, Kraft paper and board are widely diffused on the market [31]. These containers are rigid and peculiarly impermeable to oxygen and water vapour.

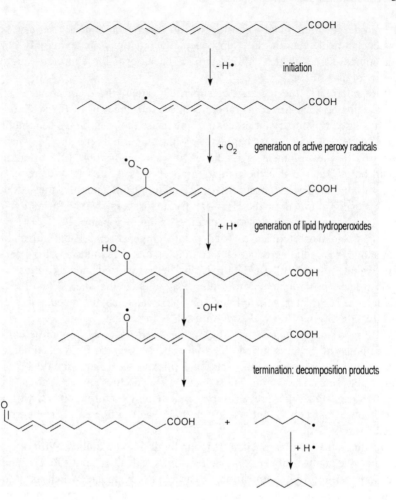

Fig. 3.1 The thermal oxidation of fatty acids. With reference to fried potato chips, the initial attack occurs in the deep-fat frying process by the formation of free radicals in presence of metal ions, heating or light exposure

However, the use of laminated films for flexible thermosealed bags is greatly appreciated: new possibilities are available with reference to the visual appearance of printed films. In addition, the improved barrier effect of metallised films increases notably the resistance of products against oxidation. One of the most appreciated supports for laminated films is polypropylene (PP). At present, main solutions appear oriented PP (OPP) when laminated with aluminium or simply coated, while uncoated OPP is not appreciated: shelf life appears sensibly reduced. For comparative purposes, it can be told that the low density polyethylene (LDPE) is not considered good for this type of application if compared with uncoated OPP [32].

Fig. 3.2 Tetrahedral food containers for fried potato chips. These packages can be realised flexible laminated films in the same way of normal bags for fried chips

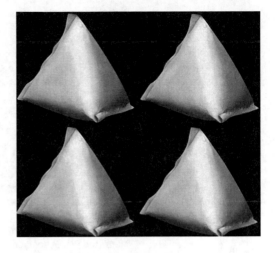

However, the use of PE and coated PE has been reported for deep-frozen and gas-packed chilled french fries (inner atmosphere: carbon dioxide and nitrogen) [33].

The present case study aims to evaluate possible differences between two similar solutions: both situations are referred to the same basic material, a laminated film for thermosealed bags.

3.4.3 Fried Potato Chips in Thermosealed Pouches: Comparison Between Two Similar Bags

The traditional flexible bag for industrial chips may be realised with different shapes, including the traditional 'vertical form-fill type' (VFF) system. This type of thermosealed bag is obtained by means of continuous, automated VFF machines with three sealings [33].

Other possible solutions may be available at present. One of these may be a tetrahedral FP (Fig. 3.2) with following features:

- Improved compactness
- Ameliorated resistance to mechanical tensions
- Enhanced protection of the contained food
- Augmented spaces for the visual communication (there are four differently printable surfaces per every FP)
- Versatility with concern to the IFP assembling and storage requirements. Different positions are available, including the innovative 'snap-fit structure' [34].

With concern to the last point, it should be clarified that chips—and other food products with low unit price—are normally packaged into soft and thin

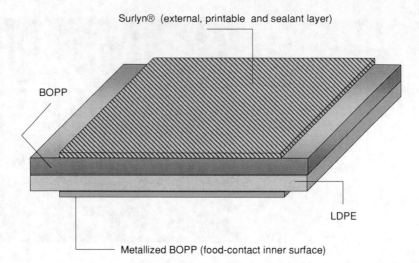

Surlyn® (external, printable and sealant layer)

BOPP

LDPE

Metallized BOPP (food-contact inner surface)

Fig. 3.3 A typical multi-layered structure for potato chip bags. The food-contact surface is metallised bi-oriented polypropylene (*metallised BOPP*); middle layers are low density polyethylene (*LDPE*) and biaxially oriented polypropylene (*BOPP*). The external, printable and sealable layer is an ethylene copolymer, Surlyn®

aluminium-made envelopes; this IFP is not requested to have excellent mechanical resistances.

Finally, the transport of tetrahedral IFP is made easier and economically convenient by means of an SRP system.

Anyway, traditional pouches and tetrahedral packages can be realised with the same film (Fig. 3.3). The food-contact surface may be metallised bi-oriented polypropylene, also named BOPP; middle layers can be low density polyethylene (LDPE) and biaxially oriented polypropylene (BOPP). Finally, external, printable and sealable layers are generally ethylene co-polymers like Surlyn® [35]. However, other solutions are available [36].

For example, the following sequences may be offered (excluding adhesive products like polyethylene amines):

1. Outermost (external) layer: transparent nylon, polyester, cellophane or polypropylene
2. Second layer: coextruded coloured or clear polyethylene and ethylene acrylic acid copolymer
3. Middle layer: aluminium foil
4. Innermost layer (sealable): heat sealable polyolefins [37].

The consumer can recognise and classify the product 'at first sight'. Above mentioned printing inks are generally formulated with organic or inorganic pigments (Sect. 2.2.5.4).

By a general viewpoint, the comparison between the two packaging solutions appears to highlight three basic elements:

- The dimension of the final IFP
- The different encumbrance of the packaged product when assembled in secondary packaging units or into multi-IFP cartons
- The quantity of packaged chip pieces into a single IFP
- Possible differences with relation to mechanical resistances and safety risks.

These features have to be discussed with physicochemical risks and failures.

3.4.4 Fried Potato Chips in Different Thermosealed Pouches: Risks and Advantages

3.4.4.1 Dimension of the Final IFP

The problem of sizes is the first factor for packaging designers and food technologists. At present, it may be inferred that the higher the possible number of available dimensions of the final IFP, the lower the number of commercially available destinations for the same product. In fact, extended sizes are surely related to notable amounts of packaged chips: as a consequence, the destination of the final IFP is mainly connected with the selling point (mass retailers, little supermarkets, etc.).

On the other hand, the problem of sizes is necessarily connected with two aspects of the primary FP: the amount of packaged foods and the encumbrance of the final IFP into secondary containers.

On these bases, it can be anticipated now that the traditional bag for fried potato chips seems to offer various options in comparison with the tetrahedral system. In fact, the classic VFF shape can contain 50, 100 or 1,000 gms of 1.5 gms-potato chip pieces per single IFP.

On the other hand, the tetrahedral FP appears fit for limited weights and dimensions because of the possible damage of the whole IFP structure under pressure. The number of sealed edges in tetrahedral IFP could be seen as a disadvantage when the packaged product is not located into pre-designed secondary containers such as SRP: 'n' corners may be 'n' weak points if the package is compressed. As a result, the traditional bag seems a logical choice for high-sized products.

3.4.4.2 Encumbrance of the Packaged Product

As above mentioned, the problem of mechanical resistances to pressure is important when speaking of flexible bags. This problem could be easily solved in both examined solutions. However, it has to be considered that:

- The traditional VFF bag is normally subjected to weak or heavy pressure when packaged in secondary packaging units such as the normal cardboard box. Because of the necessity of avoiding damages to highly-damageable flexible containers, the box should be resistant enough. However, the final opening and the displacement of bags on shelves may be difficult
- The above mentioned barrier effect of traditional bags has to be 'helped' with adequate logistic solutions. The assembling of 'n' IFP in a secondary packaging unit is requested because of the necessity of insulating the primary packaging and the contained food by the external atmosphere. This concept means that the combined effect of environmental moisture, light exposure and heating can be limited with the assembling of traditional bags into boxes
- The tetrahedral solution has a distinctive advantage if compared with the traditional VFF bag. In fact, the chosen shape of the final IFP appears directly correlated with the assembling of 'n' different IFP in a dedicated SRP. This secondary packaging is designed to be opened, placed on shelves and used as a display for IFP. Should SRP be used, it could be affirmed that the main risk of tetrahedral containers—the supposed fragileness on corners—may be avoided completely. On the other hand, the placement of 'n' different IFP in a predetermined order allows the easy preservation of foods against external agents. The sum of 'n' assembled IFP is substantially similar to a single macro-IFP with reduced exposition to heating, moisture, light rays and the consequent limitation of physicochemical risks
- As a clear result, the encumbrance of tetrahedral IFP should be reduced when these packaged products are assembled into dedicated SRP. This aspect should be evaluated when speaking of shelf life enhancement.

3.4.4.3 Amount of Packaged Chip Pieces into a Single IFP

The amount of sliced pieces into a single bag or a tetrahedral IFP is connected with other factors. Actually, the main aspect should concern shelf life and food safety. As a consequence, it should be affirmed that the best solution allows the easy and enhanced preservation and protection of the final IFP. On these bases, traditional bags appear to be fit for different sizes, dimensions and logistic systems while tetrahedral containers seem to be very helpful if correlated with SRP solutions, with improved performances. The problem of the amount of foods into a single container is directly correlated to dimensions; however, this factor can influence indirectly the speed of the chemical oxidation on sliced pieces. In fact, the higher the superficial area of exposed fried potato chips, the higher oxidation rates and the consequent production of off-flavours. As a result, the best strategy should always contrast rancidity by means of:

- The augment of weights for single piece (in other words: the reduction of thicknesses and related superficial areas), and
- The reduction of the inner oxygen into IFP.

With reference to the first problem, the thickness and related dimensions of sliced pieces may be difficultly manageable at present. For this reason, food technologists should aim to the concomitant reduction of inner volumetric capacities (sizes) and the augment of packaged products into a single FP. On these bases, traditional bags appear to allow a limited empty space while tetrahedral systems seem to reduce the possibility of entering foreign gases in favour of more abundant chips, in spite of the flexibility of the container. In addition, the weak point of every thermosealed packaging is correlated to the extension of sealings: related lengths might be lower in tetrahedral bags because of minor sizes.

3.4.5 Possible Differences with Relation to Mechanical Resistances and Safety Risks

The particular shape of the primary FP is shared with composite packages for different products: milk, frozen vegetables and so on [18]. Actually, basic supports can be different; however, the common point is always the possibility of enhancing the mechanical performance of the final container with good geometrical shapes, best available supports (the inner layer of every composite package) and the use of reliable thermosealing technologies [2]. When speaking of IFP, mechanical resistances are indirectly enhanced by means of adequate SRP solutions. With relation to traditional bags, the resistance is mainly based on the strength and the reliability of sealings.

Unfortunately, sealed areas seem the real weak point of flexible bags: should the sealing be inefficient or partial, the packaged food would be exposed to external agents with the augment of rancidity and possible safety risks.

Moreover, peculiar failures can be correlated to both types of laminated flexible bags. The contamination of packaged products by plasticisers such as phthalates is widely known [5, 18]. Plasticising agents promote the adhesion of different thin layers in laminated packaging films. With reference to packages for fried chips, the adhesion between printing inks and supports has to be ameliorated. As a result, the flexibility and the wrinkle resistance should be enhanced [26]. It may be reported that plasticisers can migrate into packed foods in spite of their use on the outer surface of laminated packages [26]. This defect is a microscopic set-off phenomenon, similarly to the macroscopic 'ghosting effect' [18].

Other food safety failures can be summarised as follows:

- Micro scratches
- Different flexibility of separated materials and consequent wrinkles (sealed areas, corners)
- Insufficient adhesion between different film layers because of the incorrect adhesion
- Incorporation of residual food fractions into the thermosealed closure with defective thermosealing, possible micro holes, anomalous fermentations and off-flavours.

As a consequence, the success of traditional bags and tetrahedral systems is always decided on the basis of these factors:

(1) Limitation of the number of IFP (influence on rancidity and consequent sensorial failures). Tetrahedral packages seem to favour this aspect but traditional bags may appear more versatile
(2) Limitation of the inner atmosphere (influence on rancidity and consequent sensorial failures). Tetrahedral packages seem to favour this aspect
(3) Excellent sealing (influence on rancidity and consequent sensorial failures; enhancement of mechanical properties). No differences between the two solutions
(4) Reduction of sealed areas (influence on rancidity and consequent sensorial failures; enhancement of mechanical properties). Tetrahedral packages seem to favour this aspect.

The balance between these properties can favour the progressive rancidity of fatty acids and other compounds in fried potato chips with the consequent emission of off-flavours.

Another reflection should be made with concern to the simple disposition of IFP into SRP. Indeed, one of possible worries for designers is the possibility of IFP damages because of incorrect SRP manufacturing during transportation and storage steps. In this case, the disposition of IFP into the proposed SRP appears reliable if all IFP can be acceptably placed into the secondary packaging. Apparently, the ample opening space of SRP does not require the excessive use of glues or similar adhesive products for assembling purposes. Probably, IFP will not suffer the following damages:

- Contact with residues of adhesive agents and partially active particles such carboxymethylcellulose, modified resins, dextrines
- Perforations by sharp structures or rivulets of used glues [18].

Secondly, the 'advertising' function should require remarkable and brilliant dyes such as monochromatic inks for generic SRP containers. These products can be formulated with organic dyes because of the excellent hue (Sect. 2.2.5.4).

Otherwise, the choice of inorganic pigments can be justified when SRP have to be stored under specific conditions: the exposure to UV rays might diminish the colorimetric tint of blue colours during extended temporal periods (Sect. 2.2.5.4).

In addition, high costs and the relative low light solidity of organic pigments may be crucial. Finally, the higher the physical adsorption of energy by means of light exposure, the higher the local amount of kinetically-enhanced chemical reactions including oxidation. For this reason, the choice of printing inks should be carefully evaluated with relation to the nature of the printed IFP and logistic destinations.

The evolution of transportation and logistics has surely influenced physical and ergonomic features of modern packages (primary, secondary and tertiary). In addition, the distribution management of different commodities can be easily monitored by means of innovative technologies. Intelligent packaging devices (Sects. 2.2.5.4 and 3.3) are the most important evolution of these systems [20].

At present, 'smart' packaging may be subdivided in two categories:

- Monitoring systems: they can give reliable interpretations of the interaction between the packaged food and external or inner agents (in the first situation, FP corresponds to the basic interface; in the second situation, the IFP is ideally separated from the external environment). Generally, monitoring devices are thermal indicators, gas detectors, biosensors, etc
- Monitoring and transmitting packaging systems: these objects are specifically designed to integrate the main monitoring function (of packaged foods) with the management of different IFP unities within a specified space (warehouse, trucks, cargos, etc.).

The second category—RFID systems—has been described in Sect. 3.3. The innovation is related to the continuous and reliable traceability of food and beverage products within extended spaces. Additionally, the monitoring function can be easily carried out on-site and off-site with evident advantages in terms of logistic management and anti-falsification or 'food defence', according to current quality management standards such as International Featured Standards (IFS) Food, version 6 [38, 39].

The category of RFID systems and similar devices is not directly correlated to food safety and chemical modifications of IFP and packaged foods. However, the reliability of official analyses and reports is dependent on the reliability and the demonstration of good storage conditions. As a result, the most part of mass retailers are focused on the problem of traceability. Consequently, this book should note at least the existence and the importance of these devices [40].

3.5 Usage Requirements

The rapid evolution of food consumption and correlated life styles has transformed the original role of FP. One of new features is the possibility of using food container as cooking, heating or cooling systems [41]. Actually, the diversification of different food products implies the similar and inevitable categorisation of FP with reference to these innovations: there are many possible examples for self-heating packaging or self-cooling packaging [19].

On the other side, the 'digital era' has implicitly but urgently forced FP and IFP designers to create new 'information technology' (IT) applications and physical supports for different foods, products and IT systems. The result is the interaction between the 'passive' IFP and the 'active' consumer by means of so-called 'social networks' and modern communication media: personal computers, smartphones, tablets, etc. Naturally, the digital flow of information has to be conveyed by means of wireless or physically connected internet networks. On these bases, the consumer can interact with IFP and FP with reference to food safety, chemistry, hygiene and environmental topics [42], and all consumers can observe and directly evaluate the evolution of FP towards the idea of 'smart packaging' devices (Sect. 2.2.5.4).

As above mentioned, usage requirements are related to different factors:

- The need of dosing systems, reliable closures, easy-open devices
- The creation of 'hybrid' package with (a) basic functions of simple packaging and (b) features of normal kitchen tools for cooking or instant refrigeration (household applications)
- The transformation of IFP in self-explaining products by means of digital technologies or physicochemical reactions.

The nature of IP solutions is still to be investigated: these systems are generally simple components. The transmission and the communication of basic information about RSL can be obtained by means of simple colorimetric variations; these changes may be interpreted and analysed with digital systems [5].

Another important challenge is the comparison between the packaged food and the IP system. In fact, every intelligent device is designed with the aim of making evident chemical, physical and textural modifications of the packaged (and often 'hidden') food. This function can be obtained only when IP mimes effectively one or more chemical or microbiological transformations of the packaged food (in the same storage condition). The design of adequate and reliable 'replica' indicators may be helpful [20].

Anyway, the interpretation of colours and other macroscopic variations has to be easily made by normal users without need of intermediary agents. This specific requirement can surely influence—and restrict—the choice of chemical principles and materials for IP systems because of two important factors. First of all, intelligent devices should be formulated with food-grade chemical intermediates or substances (otherwise, concerns of food contamination could occur).

In addition, used chemical intermediates, substances, pigments and materials (example: glass-like plastic windows for 'bull's eye' systems) have to make immediately evident all possible colorimetric or sensorial variations.

Therefore, FP can become the first example of self-explaining packaging for food consumers [43]. The importance of ergonomics and the perception of FM, IFP distributors and final consumers are fundamental: only selected chemicals can allow the transformation of the original design concept by means of the synergy between shape and aesthetics [44]. On a practical level, a specific case history can be analysed.

An interesting case study can be examined with relation to bottled red wines.

3.5.1 Food Product: Bottled Red Wine
in Asymmetrical-Shaped Bottles

Red wines are subjected to important modifications of chemical and physical profiles during their storage. Many chemical parameters may vary during time, depending on the previous method of vinification and the consequent type of desired product. For example, white wines can be classified by means of the peculiar phenolic composition: phenols can reflect the origin of grapes, growing conditions and vinification techniques [45]. In addition, they have been recognised to have an important role with relation to UV protection, disease resistance and pigmentation [46]. With specific relation to wines, the importance of phenols, phenolic acids, flavonoids, hydroxycinnamates and gallic acid is notable. Phenolic compounds include different flavonoids: for example, the flavan-3-ols (+)-catechin and (−)-epicatechin; various conjugates of flavonols, quercetin and myricetin; different anthocyanins including malvidin-3-O-glucoside [46]. Actually, there are also nonflavonoid substances: C6–C1 hydroxybenzoic acids; gallic and ellagic acids; C6–C3 hydroxycinnamates; caffeic, caftaric and p-coumaric acids; resveratrol (3,5,4′-tryhydroxystylbene) and its olygomers and glucosides [46, 47].

Chromatographic methods may detect these chemicals [45]. Hydroxycinnamates are well known for their oxidability and their role as browning precursors in white wines: trans- and cis-hydroxycinnamic acids are very important. In addition, the so-called non-enzymatic browning may be mentioned when the progressive browning and the development of off-flavours are demonstrated in wines. These chemical reactions are also known as 'Maillard reactions': this name is currently used to indicate the initial reaction of aldehyde groups in reducing sugars with free amino groups of amino acids. The production of intermediates such as acetol, diacetyl, furfuraldehyde, pyruvaldehyde, etc., is not 'the end' of the pathway: these molecules can still turn into brown melanoide-type macromolecules by reaction with amines [48]. Anyway, the importance of Maillard reactions in wines may be reduced sensibly by the use of sulphur dioxide as a reliable antioxidant.

The situation might appear more complex when speaking of red wines instead of white products. Actually, the pigmentation of these products and the more general modification of physicochemical features depend on winemaking techniques: length of skin contact, temperature, presence of seeds, stems and enzymes, etc. These parameters can affect the extraction of phenolics into the fermenting juice before the final bottling with the consequent modification of the antioxidant activity of wines [46].

After vinification, all wines may change their chemical profiles. This complex phenomenon, generally named 'wine ageing', is not entirely known at present depending on various factors: different climatic and ageing conditions including moisture, temperature, and pH; wood composition of ageing barrels, etc. [49]. Actually, ageing can be also noted into simple glass bottles. One of the more interesting variations appears related to the composition of anthocyanins: one of the most an important and abundant chemical is malvidin-3-O-glucoside (Fig. 3.4).

Fig. 3.4 The chemical structure of malvidin-3-*O*-glucoside. BKchem version 0.13.0, 2009 (http://bkchem.zirael.org/index.html) has been used for drawing this structure

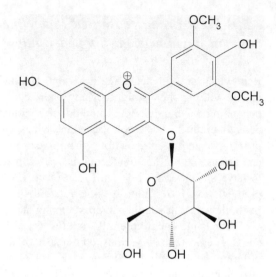

In general, acetylated and non-acetylated anthocyanins seem to decrease during time when red wines are stored in bottles because of the possible combination with tannins and the hydrolysis on non-acetylated molecules. It has been reported that the total content of anthocyanins should decrease during storage in bottles (10–15 months) because of condensation reactions with proanthocyanidins. Anyway, the importance of anthocyanins seems mainly correlated to the pigmentation of wines during ageing. In detail, anthocyanin-derived pigments are correlated to the modification of wine colours from the original purple-red to the final and desired brick-red hue [50]. It can be interesting to consider that the total pigment content in red wines may be calculated from the total area of chromatograms concerning non-fractionated samples at 520 nm. The expression of these substances may be made as malvidin-3-*O*-glucoside [50]. It has been reported that this 'target' molecule decreases normally during time when wines are aged in barrels: consequently, the highest peak of malvidin-3-*O*-glucoside is subsequently fractionated with the appearance of other peaks (new pigments and malvidin-3-*O*-glucoside derivatives). However, the final result is that the destruction of original pigments is not compensated by the production of 'new' coloured substances. This situation is well known when ageing occurs in barrels. On the other hand, bottle ageing may be more detrimental because of the increased destruction of A-type vitisins, direct condensation products and anthocyanins [50]. Could this situation be dependent on bottle types (colours, glass type, shapes, position, etc.)? This possible case study is dedicated to the synthetic explanation of the bottle ageing in a new type of designed FP.

3.5.2 Bottled Red Wines: The Horizontal Storage and Dedicated Bottles

Red wines can be packaged in different ways. Glass bottles are the most known and traditional medium because of the chemical inertness and the interesting transparency (Sect. 2.2.8.2). However, wines have to be stored at an even temperature. Sudden and/or irregular variations can cause premature ageing; in addition, wines may suffer some contraction with oxidation problems if temperatures are suddenly varied [51]. Finally, the protection against UV rays is crucial: for these reasons, glass bottles are the most attracting FP for wines; on the other side, bottled beverages have to be carefully stored.

By contrast, wines may be also packed in plastic bottles or in polycoupled packages: the known 'bag-in-box' cartons. These solutions may be seen with reduced favour by traditional consumers. Packaged wines may be preserved in non-glass containers; on the other side:

- Plastic bottles are reported to be used for airline uses (limited shelf life)
- PVC and PET containers are not universally accepted because of the possible contamination of wines (traces of solvents and plasticisers)
- 'Bag-in-box' and smaller lined cartons have good or excellent barrier effects. By contrast, the appeal of these packages may be questionable and related prices may seem unattractive.

As a result, glass bottles appear still useful in the modern industry in spite of the reduced 'stability' of wines during storage.

With reference to our case study, the comparison between old-style glass bottles and possible new shapes could be examined. The aim of designers and food technologists could be the production of attractive bottled wines with some specific advantage, particularly with concern to colours. A new shape of glass bottle can be proposed here (Fig. 3.5).

By the designer's viewpoint, the creation of particular symbols is generally focused on the communication by means of dedicated logos or printed labels. In the above mentioned situation, the design core has been substantially based on new hypotheses of shape and functions. The slanting and asymmetrical profile of glass bottles has been studied to facilitate handling and to optimise the horizontal stacking of packaging with increased stability when bottles are placed in a flat position. In addition, the central part of these FP has been designed for different labels according to communicative exigencies of awarded wine producers. As a consequence, the asymmetrical FP identifies the whole IFP among other wines in spite of the possible application of different labels. Additionally, the visual redundancy is significantly mitigated with sure advantages.

By the chemical viewpoint, the practical application of the initial designers' idea has one interesting feature. The requested asymmetry and the concomitant necessity of making easier the handling of bottles appear opposite factors in a generic design plan. Moreover, the handling should be easy and 'sure' against

Fig. 3.5 Glass bottles for red
wines, asymmetrical shape

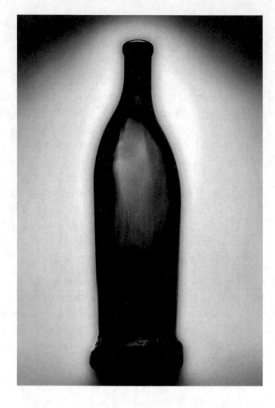

possible glides of packaging from users' and consumers' hands. The best strategy
is generally linked to the use of glass mixtures with 'exactly' determined composition. Normally, this condition should imply a dedicated manufacturing process. The multiplicity of glass powders and wrecks in glass manufacturing
determines different performances: infrangibility, opacity, transparency, roughness, necessity of superficial finishing, etc. With reference to glass bottles, a few
dedicated glass mixtures may be fit while other good chemical compositions might
be judged unreliable depending on the final application.

Chemically, the use of dedicated glass materials (with the exclusion of foreign
wrecks) means that the normal cooling of final bottles—the manufacturing step
just after the 'forming' operation (Sect. 2.2.5.4)—should be extensively prolonged
in terms of hours.

Glass networks are substantially silicon, aluminium and oxygen- based tridimensional structures with a relatively low quantity of 'empty spaces' (chemical
vacancies). Mechanical performances of the final contain can notably be modified
[52] depending on the number, the spatial disposition and the possible filling of
these vacancies by metallic ions (sodium, potassium, calcium, iron). Moreover,
different 'extraneous' metallic ions can imply enhanced properties while the
presence of other cations may worsen the performance of final products.

In addition, the tridimensional structure can be chaotic or roughly ordered depending on the time of cooling (after the fusion of powdered mixtures) and forming steps. Consequently, processing times and temperatures, chemical composition, etc., have to be preliminarily studied with the aim of assuring the physical stability of empty and full bottles. Additionally, FP could exhibit superficial defects with the necessity of finishing processes; fragileness (when infrangibility has been preliminarily requested), etc. [18].

With reference to our bottles, a possible request concerns the exterior looking. In many cases, these containers may be coloured with the addition of reliable inorganic pigments. The aim of dark tints is the filtration of UV rays by means of physical reflection. As a result, reflected light radiations give dark colours to bottles with minimal transparency. The final aim is the protection of bottled wines against UV rays because of the possible and enhanced oxidation of ascorbic acid, 3-mercaptohexanol and other oxidable compounds [53]. In addition, new wine tints can be obtained: anthocyanin–flavanol associations have been studied in recent years because of the production of derivatives in flavylium form during wine aging [54].

The practical application of the asymmetrical shape may be recommended on condition that the stability of red wines remains assured if compared with 'normal' packages. In other words, colorimetric tints of red wines should not be affected negatively by the new bottle type.

At present, it can be assumed that the visual appearance of bottled wines is not worsened when asymmetrical bottles are used. In particular, food technologists could have some doubt with relation to the horizontal position of bottles during storage. However, there are not evidences that the horizontal ageing into transparent and asymmetrical bottles may effectively reduce the total pigment quantity and the resulting tint of red wines in comparison with traditional bottles.

At present, the only difference between conventional and horizontal storage might be correlated with the permeability of closures to oxygen, on condition that remaining storage conditions are constant (temperature, environmental moisture, absence of light and dissolved catalysing metal ions in wines, etc.). The choice of closures appears crucial because of the main role of oxygen. Permeability to oxygen is optimal when synthetic closures are applied to glass bottles, while screw caps and 'technical' corks seem the best choice [55]. Anyway, it has been also reported that wine ageing by oxidation is clearly independent on the position of bottles during storage, in spite of the problem of headspaces and the possible contact between closures and bottled wines. In addition, several studies on white wines have been carried out until 24 months by storing bottled wines in the horizontal position instead of the vertical position, assuming that this system is quite challenging.

The main problem appears always related to the synthetic or conventional closure: screw caps are described as able to reduce 'rotten egg' or 'putrefaction' smells because of the production of hydrogen sulphide [55]. As a consequence, the asymmetrical bottle does not seem to have detrimental effects on sensorial features of red wines if compared with other glass containers for 'normal' storage. With the exception of this aspect, it can be assumed that the only difference between traditional and asymmetrical bottles concerns only marketing purposes without excessive influence on chemical and physical profiles of wines.

Colours may be measured in different ways. Generally, spectrophotometric methods are used [56] because of the reliability of obtained results. The redox reaction of phenolic compounds with the phosphomolybdicphosphotungstic acid (*Folin–Ciocalteu* reagent) is used: as a result, a blue-coloured complex is produced in alkaline solutions. The quantitative amount of this complex is measured at 765 nm. In addition, anthocyanins can be evaluated and expressed as malvidin-3-*O*-glucoside equivalents at 540 nm [56]. Another strategy is the colour and hue analysis by direct measurement of wine samples at wavelengths of 420, 520 and 620 nm. Alternatively, the acquisition and the colorimetric analysis of digital images are recommended [5].

With relation to bottled wines and similar beverages, the application of printed labels is normally accepted. This traditional practice may be useful because of the introduction of 'smart' packaging devices (Sect. 2.2.5.4). In fact, the main function of these systems is strictly correlated to the flow of visual information: consequently, IP devices may ameliorate usage performances of the whole IFP.

Technically, smart packaging systems can interact with external or inner agents at the same time. The first sub-class is represented by NTI and TTI (Sect. 3.3): they can give visible information related to food hygiene, safety and residual shelf life to consumers and warehouse operators. In detail, the information is supplied as:

(1) Demonstration of FP exposure to excessive thermal values, without possibility of time or temperature recording (used system: NTI)
(2) Results of thermal variations by means of chemical or physical modifications (used system: TTI).

Similarly, the physical protection is communicated and demonstrated by means of 'leakage' indicators (Sects. 2.2.5.4 and 3.3): these IP devices can modify their aspect if FP are improperly altered or have suffered mechanical stress. Other interesting IP systems are freshness indicators (Sects. 2.2.5.4 and 3.3), which show the presumptive maturation of packaged foods, usually fruits and vegetables: the key is the chemical interaction between the intelligent support (chemical substances) and emitted gaseous compounds by food surfaces.

On the other side, active packages can interact with foods for enhancing RSL values. Maybe most known types are 'scavenger' systems. These devices can absorb peculiar molecules into IFP avoiding excessive oxidation, colorimetric variations, high respiration rates, etc. Usually, most known and important components for the production of scavenger packaging are inorganic compounds. Depending on the specific target, different substances can be used [15]:

• For oxygen scavengers: ferrous compounds, organometallic scavengers, cathecol, glucose oxidase, ascorbic acid, ethanol oxidase, oxidable resins with metallic catalysers

- For ethylene scavengers: potassium permanganate on solid supports, activated carbon
- For moisture scavengers: glycerol, silica gel, polyacrilamide, mineral clays.

3.6 Disposal Requirements

The disposal of FP is seemingly a simple operation. However, environmental factors and the scarcity of determined raw materials for FP productions have significantly modified the common opinion of consumers concerning food packaging wastes; so new growing needs are affecting FP design from both quantitative and qualitative points of view.

As a result, FP designers aim to reduce intrinsic and critical points of current packaging by means of following strategies [53]:

- Reduction of sizes, in terms of volumetric capacity
- Reduction of thicknesses, where possible: reliable materials are needed [17] but the related availability can often become a difficult problem in many geographical areas
- Use of raw materials with high recycling yields (aluminium alloys, polyethylene, etc.) and low adsorption rates with reference to water (hydrophilicity may reduce recycling yields)
- Reduction of 'extraneous' but necessary additives for FP production (adhesive products for paper and board boxes, composite packaging; persistent and thermally modifiable pigments; etc.) with the aim of making easier waste collection and recycling processes [13]
- Proposal of mono-material FP in comparison with multi-material FP (example: simple paper boxes instead of composite materials).

On these bases, the design of environmentally sustainable FP has to take into account the choice of reliable and cheap materials. On the other side, the clear invitation to the disposal of packaging for subsequent recycling has to be planned by means of reliable messages and advices on packaging [57]. Two factors have to be taken into account: (a) chemical features of employed FP materials and (b) the absence—or possibility of chemical interactions—between foods and packaging.

References

1. Volli U (2012) Semiotica Della Pubblicità. Laterza, Roma
2. Piergiovanni L, Limbo S (2010) Materiali, Tecnologie E Qualità Degli Alimenti. Springer, Milan
3. Bucchetti V (2007) Packaging Contro. Verso, Dativo, Milan

4. Barbero S, Pereno A, Tamborrini P (2011) Qualitative/quantitative cross analysis to design eco-pack. In: Castillo L, Guedes M, Franklin W (eds) Proceedings of the 3rd international symposium on sustainable design (III ISSD), Recife, Sept 2011. Editora Universitària UFPE, pp 105–115
5. Parisi S (2013) Food industry and packaging materials—performance-oriented guidelines for users. Smithers Rapra Technology, Shawbury
6. Germak C (2008) Man at the centre of the project. Allemandi, Torino
7. Shinkman M, Lewis P (2008) Rich pickings, opportunities in South-east Asia's emerging markets. Atradius Credit Insurance NV and The Economist Intelligence Unit, NY, p 15. http://www.asia-now.com/files/ideas/Rich%20pickings%20Opportunities%20in%20South%20East%20Asia's%20emerging%20markets.pdf. Accessed 28 Jan 2014
8. Heskett J (2005) Design a very short introduction. Oxford University Press, Oxford
9. Marsh K, Bugusu B (2007) Food packaging—roles, materials, and environmental issues. J Food Sci 72(3):39–55. doi:10.1111/j.1750-3841.2007.00301.x
10. Vollmer A, Biedermann M, Grundböck F, Ingenhoff J-E, Biedermann-Brem S, Altkofer W, Grob K (2011) Migration of mineral oil from printed paperboard into dry foods: survey of the German market. Eur Food Res Technol 232:175–182. doi:10.1007/s00217-010-1376-6
11. Kernoghan N (2012) Mineral oil in recycled paper and board packaging. Smithers Pira. https://www.smitherspira.com/testing/food-contact/news-free-webinar-mineral-oil-in-recycled-paper-and-board-packaging.aspx. Accessed 11 Oct 2013
12. Codex Alimentarius Commission (1995) Codex general standard for food additives, last revision 2013. Codex Alimentarius—International Food Standards. http://www.codexalimentarius.net/gsfaonline/docs/CXS_192e.pdf. Accessed 18 Oct 2013
13. Bozzola M (ed) (2011) EasyEATING. Sustainable paper packaging for traditional produce, Dativo, Milan
14. Ottaviani F (2002) Il metodo HACCP (Hazard Analysis and Critical Control Points). In: Andreis G, Ottaviani F (eds) Manuale di sicurezza degli alimenti. Principi di ecologia microbica e di legislazione applicati alla produzione alimentare. Oxoid S.p.A., G. Milanese, Milan
15. Micali M, Parisi S, Minutoli E, Delia S, Laganà P (2009) Alimenti confezionati e atmosfera modificata. Caratteristiche basilari, nuove procedure, applicazioni pratiche. Ind Aliment 489:35–43
16. Pereno A (2012) Tra comunicazione e prodotto: il packaging. In: Tamborrini P, Barbero S (eds) Il Fare Ecologico. Il prodotto industriale e i suoi requisiti ambientali, Edizione Ambiente, Milano, pp 88–90
17. Boylston S (2009) Designing sustainable packaging. Laurence King Publishing Ltd., London
18. Parisi S (2012) Food packaging and food alterations: the user-oriented approach. Smithers Rapra Technology, Shawbury
19. Parisi S (2004) Alterazioni in Imballaggi Metallici Termicamente Processati. Gulotta Press, Palermo
20. Parisi S (2009) Intelligent packaging for the food industry. In: Carter EJ (ed) Polymer electronics—a flexible technology. Smithers Rapra Technology Ltd, Shawbury
21. Ceppa C, Fassio F, Marino G (2008) Food-pack guidelines. Time & Mind, Torino
22. Yam KL, Takhistov PT, Miltz J (2005) Intelligent packaging: concepts and applications. J Food Sci 70(1):1–10. doi:10.1111/j.1365-2621.2005.tb09052.x
23. De Kruijf N, van Beest M, Rijk R, Sipiläinen-Malm T, Paseiro Losada P, De Meuleunaer B (2002) Active and intelligent packaging: applications and regulatory aspects. Food Addit Contam 19(Suppl):144–162. doi:10.1080/02652030110072722
24. Soroka W (2003) Packaging technology. Italian Institute of Packaging, Milan
25. Parisi S (2002) I fondamenti di calcolo della data di scadenza degli alimenti: principi ed applicazioni. Ind Aliment 417:905–919
26. Brown H, Williams J (2003) Packaged product quality and shelf life. In: Coles R, McDowell D, Kirwan MJ (eds) Food packaging technology. Blackwell Publishing Ltd, Oxford

27. Man YC, Tan CP (1999) Effects of natural and synthetic antioxidants on changes in refined, bleached, and deodorized palm olein during deep-fat frying of potato chips. J Am Oil Chem Soc 76(3):331–339. doi:10.1007/s11746-999-0240-y

28. Fuller G, Guadagni DG, Weaver ML, Notter G, Horvat RJ (1971) Evaluation of oleic safflower oil in frying of potato chips. J Food Sci 36(1):43–44. doi:10.1111/j.1365-2621.1971.tb02028.x

29. Mariod A, Matthaus B, Eichner K, Hussein IH (2006) Frying quality and oxidative stability of two unconventional oils. J Am Oil Chem Soc 83(6):529–538. doi:10.1007/s11746-006-1236-5

30. Shahidi F, Wanasundara UN (2002) Methods for measuring oxidative rancidity in fats and oils. In: Akon CC, Min DB (eds) Food lipids: chemistry, nutrition and biotechnology, pp 387–403

31. Baur FJ (1970) Packaging of chip-type snack food products. US Patent 3,498,798, 3 Mar 1970

32. Kirwan MJ, Strawbridge JW (2003) Plastics in food packaging. In: Coles R, McDowell D, Kirwan MJ (eds) Food packaging technology. Blackwell Publishing Ltd, Oxford

33. Keijbets MJH (2001) Improving product quality. The manufacture of pre-fried potato products. In: Rossell JB (ed) Frying: improving quality, vol 56. Woodhead Publishing, Cambridge, pp 195–214

34. Li H, Jin K, He B, Chen Y (2012) Hollow structure snap-fit design embedded with shape memory polymer sheet. CIRP Ann Manuf Technol 61(1):31–34. doi:10.1016/j.cirp.2012.03.110

35. Jansen AN, Amine K, Newman AE, Vissers DR, Henriksen GL (2002) Low-cost, flexible battery packaging materials. JOM 54(3):29–32. doi:10.1007/BF02822616

36. Butler TI, Morris BA (2009) PE based multilayer film structures. In: Wagner JR Jr (ed) Multilayer flexible packaging: technology and applications for the food, personal care, and over-the-counter pharmaceutical industries. Elsevier, Amsterdam, pp 205–230

37. Snow JE (1981) Laminated packaging material. US Patent 4,363,841, 14 Dec 1982

38. Unander T, Nilsson H-E (2011) Evaluation of RFID based sensor platform for packaging surveillance applications. In: 2011 IEEE international conference on RFID-technologies and applications, RFID-TA 2011, art. no. 6068611, pp 27–31

39. Schulze H, Albersmeier F, Gawron JC, Spiller A, Theuvsen L (2008) Heterogeneity in the evaluation of quality assurance systems: The International Food Standard (IFS) in European Agribusiness. Int Food Agribus Manag Rev 11(3):99–139

40. Stilo A, Parisi S, Delia S, Anastasi F, Bruno G, Laganà P (2009) La Sicurezza Alimentare in Europa: confronto tra il 'Pacchetto Igiene' e gli Standard British Retail Consortium (BRC) ed International Food Standard (IFS). Ann Ig 21(4):387–401

41. Hartmann C, Dohle S, Siegrist M (2013) Importance of cooking skills for balanced food choices. Appetite 65(1):125–131. doi:10.1016/j.appet.2013.01.016

42. Lowe B, de Souza-Monteiro DM, Fraser I (2013) Nutritional labelling information: utilisation of new technologies. J Mark Manag 29(11–12):1337–1366. doi:10.1080/0267257X.2013.798673

43. Ciravegna E (2010) La Qualità Del Packaging. Franco Angeli, Milano

44. Tosi F (2005) Ergonomia, Progetto, Prodotto. Franco Angeli, Milan

45. Betés-Saura C, Andrés-Lacueva C, Lamuela-Raventós RM (1996) Phenolics in white free run juices and wines from Penedès by high-performance liquid chromatography: changes during vinification. J Agric Food Chem 44(10):3040–3046. doi:10.1021/jf9601628

46. Burns J, Gardner PT, Matthews D, Duthie GG, Lean J, Crozier A (2001) Extraction of phenolics and changes in antioxidant activity of red wines during vinification. J Agric Food Chem 49(12):5797–5808. doi:10.1021/jf010682p

47. Mattivi F, Reniero F, Korhammer S (1995) Isolation, characterization, and evolution in red wine vinification of resveratrol monomers. J Agric Food Chem 43(7):1820–1823. doi:10.1021/jf00055a013

48. Tucker GS (2003) Food biodeterioration and methods of preservation. In: Coles R, McDowell D, Kirwan MJ (eds) Food packaging technology. Blackwell Publishing Ltd, Oxford, pp 32–64

49. Del Alamo Sanza M, Nevares Domínguez I (2006) Wine aging in bottle from artificial systems (staves and chips) and oak woods: Anthocyanin composition. Anal Chim Acta 563(1):255–263. doi:10.1016/j.aca.2005.11.030
50. Alcalde-Eon C, Escribano-Bailón MT, Santos-Buelga C, Rivas-Gonzalo JC (2006) Changes in the detailed pigment composition of red wine during maturity and ageing: a comprehensive study. Anal Chim Acta 563(1):238–254. doi:10.1016/j.aca.2005.11.028
51. Ranken MD, Baker CG, Kill RC (eds.) (1997) Fats and fatty foods. In: Ranken MD, Baker CG, Kill RC (eds) Food Industries manual, Springer, New York, pp 272–315. doi: 10.1007/978-1-4613-1129-4_8
52. Yamato Y (1991) Glass containers. In: Kadoya T (ed) Food packaging. Academic Press, San Diego
53. Ugliano M, Kwiatkowski M, Vidal S, Capone D, Siebert T, Dieval JB, Aagaard O, Waters EJ (2011) Evolution of 3-Mercaptohexanol, hydrogen Sulfide, and methyl mercaptan during bottle storage of sauvignon blanc wines. Effect of glutathione, copper, oxygen exposure, and closure-derived oxygen. J Agric Food Chem 59(6):2564–2572. doi:10.1021/jf1043585
54. Dias DA, Clark AC, Smith TA, Ghiggino KP, Scollary GR (2013) Wine bottle colour and oxidative spoilage: whole bottle light exposure experiments under controlled and uncontrolled temperature conditions. Food Chem 138(4):2451–2459. doi:10.1016/j.foodchem.2012.12.024
55. Lopes P, Saucier C, Teissedre PL, Glories Y (2006) Impact of storage position on oxygen ingress through different closures into wine bottles. J Agric Food Chem 54(18):6741–6746. doi:10.1021/jf0614239
56. Ivanova V, Dörnyei Á, Márk L, Vojnoski B, Stafilov T, Stefova M, Kilár F (2011) Polyphenolic content of Vranec wines produced by different vinification conditions. Food Chem 124(1):316–325. doi:10.1016/j.foodchem.2010.06.039
57. Pereno A (2012) Tra comunicazione e prodotto: il packaging. In: Tamborrini P, Barbero S (eds) Il Fare Ecologico. Il prodotto industriale e i suoi requisiti ambientali. Edizione Ambiente, Milano, pp 88–90

Chapter 4
Packaging, A Communicative Medium

Abstract Functional features and graphic design are essential aspects of food packaging. Communicative requirements often define main features of modern packaging but, at the same time, communication strategies have to take into account technological potentialities of new packaging and the availability of raw materials. Every explicit or hidden feature of food packaging, which is part of the 'integrated food product', has to be communicated: ergonomic properties, mechanical strength, chemical properties, environmental sustainability, reusability, dietary advices, possibility of 'intelligent' applications with reference to the definition of remaining durability and the assessment of storage conditions, etc. All the above-mentioned factors are undoubtedly useful information to make the user aware, in spite of widespread disinformation.

Keywords Food packaging · Communication · Integrated food product · Information technology · User awareness · Chromatic appearance · Technological suitability

Abbreviations

ECCS	Electrolytic chromium-coated steel
FM	Food manufacturer
FP	Food packaging
FPP	Food packaging producer
IT	Information technology
IFP	Integrated food product
V	Light intensity
MBT	3-methylbut-2-ene-1-thiol
PET	Polyethylene terephthalate
RFID	Radio Frequency Identification

© The Author(s) 2014
G. Brunazzi et al., *The Importance of Packaging Design for the Chemistry of Food Products*, SpringerBriefs in Chemistry of Foods,
DOI: 10.1007/978-3-319-08452-7_4

RSL   Remaining shelf life
TFS   Tin free steel
UV   Ultraviolet
US   United States

4.1 Packaging and Communication: An Introduction

Functional features and graphic design are essential aspects of food and non-food packaging. Communicative requirements often define main features of modern packaging—materials, shape, sizes, opening systems, closures, qualitative and quantitative composition of separated components, etc. (Sect. 2.2.5).

At the same time, communication strategies have to take into account technological potentialities of new FP. In other words, communication may be essential for designers, technicians and marketing executives. However, the availability of good raw materials may become a challenging obstacle for the final realisation; moreover, packaging technologies might suggest other different and apparently non-innovative FP. For example, the 'eternal' debate between food technologists about the choice between metal cans (the 'old' can) and modern plastic packaging appears endless at present.

As a result, FP have to be self-explanatory, becoming the main vehicle of communication for users [2]. So, every explicit or 'hidden' feature of FP—part of the 'integrated food product' (IFP)—has to be communicated: ergonomic properties, mechanical strength, chemically refined superficial roughness, colorimetric performances of packaged goods, environmental sustainability, etc. All above-mentioned factors are undoubtedly useful information to make the consumer aware, in spite of widespread disinformation [3].

FP functional and technological features have to be 'translated' and communicated depending on the cultural level and knowledge of the receiver. The final user is considered the main target but other stakeholders should be considered: national and international consumer associations, official authorities for food inspection and analysis, academic groups, etc.

Moreover, FP has to communicate a specific message to targeted categories: required features, properties and every necessary requisite are effectively supplied with the specific packaged food [4, 5]. Consequently, this IFP has to appear 'exactly' the desired and researched object (persuasive message). The specificity of the whole IFP should be noted but common consumers do not seem to be aware of the difference between the packaged food and the integration between food, FP and other accessory products or services (Sect. 2.1). This clarification is important: the consumer is often considered as a 'passive' player of the food chain. But the user is actually the decision-maker of the whole process. Indeed, the perfect correspondence between the original consumption demand and the available offers is very difficult.

First of all, the visual redundancy of different but similar competitors (in the same food macro-category) on the same shelf can prevent the reliable prediction of related decisional processes. Moreover, the number of different IFP sizes is another important factor: the spreading of alternative offers can become excessive if every brand is represented by two IFP with different weights, volumes or shapes.

The success of marketing strategies could be linked to different factors: the maximisation of typologies of the same product line; the distinctiveness of peculiar IFP; the visibility of product communication; etc. Of course, the role of FP should be discussed and other persuasive factors have to be taken into account [6].

In addition, the increasing diversification of food markets has seen the proposal of various 'imitation' foods [7]. Correlated phenomena—spreading of versions and sub-versions of the same product; subdivision of traditional food categories in micro 'niches'—has also been observed and correctly interpreted in recent times [8]. The expansion of food markets should be also analysed in terms of food chemistry; moreover, other problems may be discussed and correctly highlighted. With reference to recent adulteration and fraud events, the use of food additives and chemical intermediates should be carefully investigated.

Another problem is correlated to the application of the same or similar packaging strategy to different competitors. On the one side, this behaviour is absolutely inevitable: a relatively low number of food packaging producers (FPP) are available and the amount of FP-related patents may appear insufficient.

On the other hand, this situation can determine the undeniable but 'grotesque' success of one historical and well-known brand among other competitors if every shown IFP appear really similar to one famous product [6, 9]. Unluckily, the scarcity of several raw materials (example: metallic supports, some polymeric commodity of large use) or intermediates (brilliant inks; adhesive products; etc.) for FP production may be the first cause for these situations. As a consequence, marketing issues and cost-cutting choices (ink selection, availability of materials, etc.) may influence the cognitive and perceptive capability of normal users if a determined IFP appears too similar to other brand products [10].

For example, the simple substitution of a peculiar but unavailable red ink based on toluidine red—(1Z)-1-[(4-methyl-2-nitrophenyl)hydrazinylidene] naphthalen-2-one—with different dyes and pigments like copper phthalocyanine (π form, crystalline modification, tint: reddish blue) can make the final FP design very similar to other branded packaging in which red colours may tend to blue tints [11].

4.2 Food and Communication

The communicative specificity of IPF is really notable and should be analysed by different viewpoints.

Usually the food market has been always considered as one of worst 'battle grounds' in the modern world because of three features:

- Foods and beverages are perceived by consumers as essential goods
- IFP may surely influence human health
- Packaged foods are often perceived as 'equivalent' goods by consumers because of the 'filtering' function of applied FP and related brands.

The last point is really important: consumers seem to be aware of their loss of direct perception of food quality. Moreover, eating behaviours have been radically and rapidly evolved in recent times with the consequent loss of cultural heritage in several industrialised countries: currently, we are seeing both the introduction of foreign gastronomic traditions and the partial recovery of 'ancient' culinary rituals [12, 13].

The recent mutation of dietary behaviours and the growing sedentariness in industrialised countries has profoundly influenced the food production [14]. The globalisation of food commodities should be considered: this phenomenon has been probably observed and nearly realised in the 1920s within different sectors and commodities, just before the initial fall in stock prices in the United States (US), also known as the Great Depression (1929). All these factors and the increasing urbanisation have substantially modified the world of food markets.

On the one side, the affirmation of edible products with high concentration of fats and carbohydrates if compared with proteins and vegetable fibres; on the other hand, the consequent countertrend has encouraged the commercialisation of breakfast foods with notable amounts of vegetable fibres and mineral substances [15, 16]. For example, 'all-bran' products and other breakfast cereals have a peculiar chemical composition: most important analytes are generally:

- Carbohydrates (starch and sugars)
- Dietary fibres
- Proteins
- Mineral elements like calcium, magnesium and zinc (related analytical contribution to ash content is notable) [17].

With reference to new industrial foods, it could be also noted that both IFP classes—general fatty or soft snacks on the one side, healthy and 'light' cereals on the other hand—appear to be packaged with similar or homogeneous FP. Usually, these are paper and board boxes or composite packaging. However, the main difference is represented by the peculiar brand and the visual communication: consequently, printed messages should be clear and vivid. In addition, packaged foods should be depicted with brilliant colours. These features require the careful choice of printing techniques, good base and reliable inks (Sect. 2.2.5.4).

In addition, the increasing trend in favour of ready-to-eat foods has to be highlighted, as recently reported: with exclusive reference to US, 77 % of consumers prefer this type of product instead of traditional foods [18]. However, the natural reaction to ready-to-eat products can be easily observed and analysed: the defence and promotion of natural (unpackaged, unprocessed) foods and the attention to 'fair trade' products can persuade a significant portion of people to abandon 'one-stop' shopping practices [19].

Both tendencies have to be supported from the visual viewpoint by means of visible and printed information, logos and images. Of course, FP have to be the real mediator between food and 'user' [20, 21].

Finally, the recent evolution of social networks has implicitly proposed new communicative functions for FP, with the consequent modification of packaging roles as advertising media [4]: the digital sharing of information can concern nutritional data and other contents: pictures, recipes, culinary advices, etc. The future FP could show less printed images than usual by means of digital, free and downloadable information [22]. Indeed the new idea of 'digital' FP and the corresponding IFP cannot be realised without the necessary interconnection on the Web and physical hardware devices [23].

The above-mentioned 'sharing' phenomenon corresponds to the logical consequence of the arrival of information technology (IT) devices in the logistic world. In fact, the simple identification of IFP by means of 'Radio Frequency Identification' (RFID) systems or the easy download of digital data by means of barcode scanners have been first introduced in the distributive field.

On the other hand, IT systems may be very useful with reference to IFP and FP analysis. In detail, the food manufacturer (FM) has the right and the responsibility of checking the possible detection of chemical, physical and microbiological risks. Chemical analysis may be performed on sampled materials with destructive methods; the same thing can be affirmed when speaking of microbiological examination or mechanical testing methods. In contrast, IT technology may allow the easy, preliminary and non-destructive detection of colorimetric or textural defects of foods [24]. These failures can be related to one or more of following causes:

- Chemical reactions, including the possibility of undesired or accelerated interactions between food and FP components
- Microbiological spreading (example: occurrence of hydrolytic deamination in several foods with consequent colorimetric modification)
- Mechanical defects (example: effects of sudden bumps on external FP).

Generally, FP failures are related to packaging manufacturing. However, the IFP is the ideal and synergetic union between the edible food and the external packaging; as a result, FP defects are correlated to food failures [25]. For example, several pasteurised 'hot *chilli*' sauces may be packaged in different packaging including tin cans and flexible aluminium tubes. With reference to 'three-piece' metal cans [24], these containers can show epoxyphenolic enamels or 'golden' coatings on the inner (food-contact) side. It has been recently observed that these sauces may easily transfer their own coloured pigments to white enamels on inner surfaces. Actually, this reaction is normal and expected when speaking of white enamels for tomato sauces and similar applications [1].

In addition, the superficial coloration may be correlated with chromatic transformations of sauces during time with notable advantages when speaking of 'remaining shelf life' (RSL) assessment. However, common consumers may be alarmed: should coloured pigments and other substances (carotenoids, lycopene, etc.) be transferred and permanently released to coated surfaces? The subsequent and natural question could be: can FP enamels release its own components (titanium dioxide, other mineral substances, epoxyphenolic compounds, etc.) in exchange for 'received' pigments [26]. Obviously, this matter is not strictly dependent of FP; on the other side, inexperienced consumers may be puzzled.

4.3 Appellative Function

Currently, every IFP should allow [27, 28] the easy and rapid identification of the related food category, including brands and possible subtypes (different sizes, weights, volumetric capacities, etc.). Naturally, FP has to satisfy these 'appellative' requirements (Sect. 2.2.5). Consequently, pictures and colours are fundamental elements: should they be correctly designed, the intuitive and unconscious reference to known and well-established mental models of food products would be assured [29]. Anyway, every FP has to show the 'right' chromatic code in function of the cultural heritage of final users [2].

From the designer's viewpoint, the chromatic and printing yield is very important. This decision concerns different stakeholders: FM and FPP have to decide if a peculiar FP design may be used. A partial list of the above-mentioned food stakeholders should comprehend at least [30, 31]:

- The FM. This subject has to make clearly the final choice about different FP
- The FPP
- The producer of main FP raw materials. Depending on the final packaging, main components may be: rigid, semi-rigid or flexible plastics (polyethylene, polypropylene, polyamides, polyesters, etc.); metal supports (tin-coated steels and aluminium alloys); glass (ingredients: sand, soda ash, limestone, feldspar, recovered glass and different chemicals compounds); paper and board (by wood pulp and recovered paper), composite packages (different components)
- The manufacturer of secondary raw materials for FP. Depending on the final packaging, a long list of compounds may be considered:
- For plastic matters and composite packages: chemical solvents, coadjutants, polymerisation retardants, various pigments, prepared printing inks
- For can packaging: food-contact approved coatings, printing inks, gaskets, etc.
- For glass packages: inorganic additives for special glasses, additives for superficial finishing and patination, crown corks, plastic caps, aluminium easy-openable crown caps
- For paper and board: optical brightener agents, adhesive products, printing inks
- The FP designer. This subject has to make different proposals on the basis of available information and main requirements by FM. The initial choice will be used to produce the first prototype.

With reference to printing inks, the composition cannot exclude the use of inorganic or organic colourants (Sect. 2.2.5.4). Printing inks—ultraviolet and traditional products, depending on drying and polymerisation techniques—contain also resins, solvents and various additives [1, 33].

In detail, the presence of resins is useful for the easy and stable binding of inks to printed supports. Solvents are also necessary because of the original physical state of inks: these products are liquid with colloidal behaviour before application on surfaces, and this metastable 'structure' should be preserved until the final printing procedure. Finally, additives are useful because of the necessity of altering physical properties of produced inks depending on different applications.

The inorganic or organic composition of pigments can determine the 'light solidity' performance (resistance to chromatic alterations against the action of light) of resulting printing inks. Anyway, the lithographic composition shows clearly that deposed inks are successively protected with a transparent coating. Additionally, the plastic composition of the final coating, also named 'finishing coating', is designed with the aim of maximising the reflection of the incident light on external surfaces of caps [1, 33]. For this reason, the final closure can appear bright instead of the predictable opaque aspect of plastic-made coatings. Of course, designers want to give back the metallic brightness to the original metal support [24].

On these bases, it can be affirmed that the superficial appearance of easy-to-open aluminium caps (and normal closures) for glass bottles can be complex enough. At the same time, it should be also noted that differences in light solidity performances may be caused by improper storage. Once more, FP and related components may act as 'active' supports if food technologists want to examine them by this viewpoint.

With relation to glass bottles, it should be requested that the bottled liquid is easily visible and identifiable. Naturally, other requirements may be important: mechanical resistance, infrangibility, absence of superficial imperfections, etc. All these factors strongly depend on processing technologies—the time of gradient cooling is a critical parameter [25], but the influence of the chemical composition is notable and critical. In fact, 50 % and more of raw materials for glass bottles are constituted of recycled materials. As a consequence, the careful selection of used glass materials is absolutely needed. Otherwise, important defects can occur with exclusive concern to glass FP: superficial imperfections, difficult finishing processes, incipient ruptures, micro fractures, intermolecular tensions in the composite silicon-based matrix [24], etc.

In the above discussed situation, the required transparency has to be complete. The presence of metallic or non-metallic contaminants in little proportions could affect the chromatic yield of glass bottles with undesired effects on the whole IFP. Most known and observable defects may be judged as simple technological imperfections when referred to the unused bottle, but the detection on final IFP may be sufficient for questioning the 'technological suitability' of FP, according to European laws [12, 24].

Finally, the hygienic evaluation of bottles beverages cannot be excluded. Basically, there are several known defects for glass bottles [24, 25]:

- Micro bubbling: possible presence of micro air bubbles in glass matrices during the 'refining' step (temperature from 1,450–1,550 °C). Associated risk: glass FP can show inner fractures where micro bubbles are present. Associated causes: excessive melting times; excessive presence of molecular vacancies into glass matrices; incorrect proportion between different elements
- Inner micro fractures with possibility of superficial evidence. Associated causes: discontinuity of the chemical composition in molten glass fluids; different thermal values in the same molten fluid during cooling and shaping steps; sudden decrease of thermal values (normally, temperatures should remain between 1,000 and 1,350 °C); presence of micro air bubbles
- Superficial scratches, inner or superficial macro ruptures. Associated causes: too rapid cooling, heterogeneous composition of glass mixtures (including the presence of unfit recovered glass), superficial damages on moulds used for shaping
- Sudden fractures, superficial damages and local chromatic variations. Associated causes: incorrect chemical formulation; wrong mixture of glass components (mixing step); rheological failures; too rapid cooling; presence of micro air bubbles; cooling steps. The first of these passages is introduced by the 'cutting' of molten glass
- Sharp edges. Cause: incorrect management of coating (or shaping and glass annealing steps)
- Scraps and shivers into empty FP. Cause: incorrect management of quality control procedures
- Poor cleanliness (including deposition of stratification of calcium carbonate on wetted surfaces) and mechanical performance, for reusable glass FP only. Associated causes: incorrect washing with caustic solutions and subsequent drying; protracted contact with strong or slightly acid foods; sudden thermal shocks; accelerated 'ageing' and consequent risk of inner fractures. In fact, silica-like structures are essentially amorphous networks; they should tend to chaotic and thermodynamically favoured glassy matrices.

Actually, several different episodes may be simply defined as 'physical contamination'. For example, one of last known episodes has concerned notable amounts of Mexican beer products [24]: these beverages have been recalled from the market because of evident and visually detectable failures (dispersed glass fragments). Other situations may be caused by microbial spreading and consequent abnormal fermentation [34].

On the other hand, the different 'tint' of coloured beers into transparent bottles may be helpful when speaking of abnormal fermentations. In fact, so-called 'intelligent packaging' systems (Sect. 3.3) are explicitly designed with the aim of making evident the decay of foods by means of simple methods, including colorimetric variations. Consequently, it could be assumed that coloured beers may make evident possible food fermentations because of the notable variation of related colours. Substantially, these products may be considered 'natural intelligent systems' on condition that chromatic variations may be easily observable by means of transparent packaging. An interesting case study may concern this peculiar beverage typology in comparison with 'normal' beers.

4.3.1   Case Study. Coloured Beers in Transparent Glass Bottles

Beers are defined as alcoholic beverages brewed from germinated barley (malt), hops, yeast, and water [12]. The number of commercial beers is notable because of the peculiar process of fermentation, the choice of available raw materials on the current market and the consequent physicochemical profile: several hundreds of chemical constituents have been identified at present [35]. The chemical composition of commercial beers—*lager* beer, porter, *Obergariges Einfachbier*, stout, barley wine, brown beer, *pilsner*, weiss beer, malt liquor, light beer, etc.—is mainly dependent on the peculiar type of yeast fermentation. Carbohydrates are converted to ethanol by means of the action of selected micro organisms such as *Saccharomyces cerevisiae* [36], although different pathways may be considered and a short list of chemical compounds may be obtained at the same time. Thermal processes have to be also considered: beers are subjected to cold pasteurisation by membrane filtration with the aim of removing living bacteria from water [37].

Beers are extremely sensible to rapid oxidation processes, similarly to wines (Sect. 3.5.2): a maximum amount of 1–2 ppm is allowed for pasteurised beers [38]. For these reasons, several packaging solutions—aluminium cans above all—require adequate pressure controls for carbonated products: positive values are required, although the excessive pressure can be detrimental. Generally, a de-aeration process is required for used ingredients; moreover, low filling temperatures should be applied [39].

With concern to organoleptic defects and safety risks, bottled and canned beers appear to be questionable when following contaminants are detected [39]:

- Metal ions such as iron. Safety is compromised. In addition, off-flavours and colorimetric variations can easily occur (iron is a good catalyser). Actually, the problem is mainly correlated with canned beers in spite of the coating protection. For this reason, highly sensible wines cannot be packed in tinplate cans: when speaking of metal cans, the choice has to be obligatorily directed towards aluminium containers. Anyway, some chelating agent might be used with the aim of contrasting colorimetric modifications
- Aluminium. This metal can be naturally found in canned beers. Related failure: cloudiness.

As above displayed, the use of cans is widely diffused but several concerns may advice brewers to use other containers. Glass bottles are widely preferred for commercial beers [40]: approximately, 30 % at least of the total market of glass bottles is reported to be used for beers. Actually, some plastic application may be suggested such as coextruded polyethylene terephthalate (PET)/'diamond-like coating' bottles or polyethylene naphthalene dicarboxylate containers [41]. However, glass seems still the best choice because of the insufficient barrier effect of PET coated surfaces, in spite of the recent development of adequate oxygen scavengers.

On these bases, it can be affirmed that glass containers should preserve bottled beers for extended temporal periods. Actually, the problem of flavour and colour stability has to be carefully evaluated. Other sensorial alterations can be observed with reference to tastes, but the visibility of colours and flavours may be a critical factor before the consumption [42].

Beer aromas can be modified when carbonyls are produced in a very little amount. Generally, aldehydes and ketones can be obtained by the degradation of following substrates [42]:

(a) Amino acids. Observed reaction: Strekker degradation. Catalysing substances: melanoidins, polyphenols
(b) Alcohols. Observed reaction: photo-oxidation to aldehydes. Catalysing substances: melanoidins. Inhibition by polyphenols
(c) Fatty acids. Observed reaction: autoxidation
(d) Lipids. Observed reaction: lipolysis
(e) Generated aldehydes. Observed reactions: aldolcondensation; secondary autoxidation of long-chain unsaturated molecules
(f) Isohumulones. Observed reaction: oxidation.

The catalysing effect of temperature or light exposure is not equally demonstrated for all above mentioned reactions. Certainly, oxygen should be minimised: on the other hand, photo-oxidation and other reactions occur at the same time. As a result, the prevailing of one or another pathway is not easily demonstrable.

Anyway, one of the best known degradations in several beers concerns the production of 3-methylbut-2-ene-1-thiol from hydrogen sulphide. In addition, the same sulphur compound may be obtained from a light-activated nascent sulphydryl compound. This molecule is obtained from sulphured amino acids (example: cysteine) and isoprendiene from the 4-methyl-3-pentenoyl-side chain of *cis*- and *trans*-isohumulones. These iso-α-acid compounds (Fig. 4.1) contribute to the bitter taste of beer [42]. The photochemical reaction is radicalic and can be catalysed by riboflavin. The resulting flavour, known as 'light struck', occurs in white or very light-coloured beers and in green or colourless bottles. Actually, some situation has been also reported in brown bottles for longer storage times under light exposure [42, 43].

Several methods have been made available for the reduction of 'light struck' flavours. The absorption or the chemical binding of the photocatalyser riboflavin is recommended; other procedures suggest the use of fructosazines or the addition of 1,8-epoxy compounds to malt beverages with the aim of preventing the formation of 3-methylbut-2-ene-1-thiol (MBT) [44–46].

Anyway, the main cause for this failure is the exposure of beers to ultraviolet (UV) rays in the 350–500 nm range.

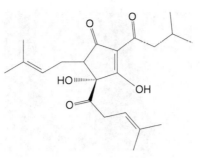

Fig. 4.1 The chemical structure of isohumulone, IUPAC name: 3,4-dihydroxy-5-(3-methylbut-2-enyl)-2-(3-methyl-1-oxobutyl)-4-(4-methyl-1-oxopent-3-enyl)-1-cyclopent-2-enone [1]. Chemical abstract service (CAS) 25522-96-7, molecular formula: C21H30O5, molecular weight: 362.46 g mol^{-1}. BKchem version 0.13.0, 2009 (http://bkchem.zirael.org/index.html) has been used for drawing this structure

The influence of the class colour of beer bottles on 'light struck' flavour is well known at present. For this reason, brown bottles are recommended if compared with green bottles because the light sensitivity of beers can be ranged between 400 and 500 nm. In fact, green glass transmits light rays between 250 and 500 nm [44, 47] while brown glass tends to cut off these radiations. Anyway, the shorter the maximum wavelength of absorbed rays, the higher the amount of produced MBT.

However, a different strategy has been recently suggested: some beer can be previously coloured with food-grade colourant substances and transparent, colourless glass bottles may be used.

On the basis of above-mentioned discussions, could food technologists compare coloured beers in transparent bottles with normal (clear) beverages in coloured (green, sky blue, red) glass containers?

4.3.1.1 Coloured Beers into Transparent Bottles: The Importance of 'Light Struck' Flavours

It should be recognised that a simple answer to the question of the last section cannot be absolute.

The suggested comparison between two different IFP has to be initially considered by the marketing viewpoint: the use of transparent bottles should reveal immediately the true colour of beers without possible errors. From the commercial viewpoint, the concept of self-displaying beers without 'masking' effects can be accepted. From the chemical viewpoint, several perplexities can be mentioned.

With concern to the question, the comparison has to be made between:

- A first choice: artificially coloured beers (sky blue, green, red tints) in association with transparent glass bottles
- A second product (Fig. 4.2): light-coloured beers in association with coloured glass bottles (sky blue, green, red tints).

Fig. 4.2 The appellative
function and packaging.
Transparent glass bottles for
coloured beverages (the
normal 'filtering' protection
of coloured glass bottles has
been transferred in the
beverage itself)

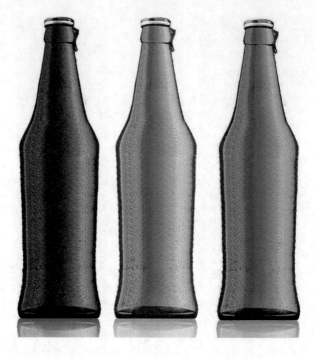

Basically, the production of MBT by photochemical reactions is function of the
following parameters:

- Concentration of sulphured amino acids (example: cysteine)
- Amount of *cis*- and *trans*-isohumulones
- Concentration of riboflavin
- Absorption of UV rays in the 350–500 nm wavelength region
- Time of exposure to UV light.

On these bases, it can be affirmed that the risk of increased failures depends
strongly from the bottled beer. UV absorption and times of exposure should be
considered in a second step.

At present, there are no available studies about the convenience of coloured
beers in transparent bottles, if compared with the traditional bottling of light-
coloured beers in coloured containers. More research is surely needed in relation to
this problem. However, it can be recognised that:

- The absorption of UV rays is favoured when transparent, blue or green bottles
  are used because of the notable or measurable transmission of high energy
  radiations between 350 and 500 nm
- By contrast, amber or brown bottles should reduce sensibly the amount of
  produced MBT: these packages are reported to have a limited absorption in the
  350–500 nm

Table 4.1 Theoretical risk by production of 3-methylbut-2-ene-1-thiol (MBT) for different beers and glass bottles

Bottled beer	Glass bottle	MBT risk (P)	Bottled beer	Glass bottle	MBT risk (P)
Brown or dark-coloured beer	Brown or dark-coloured bottle	16	Light-coloured beer	Brown or dark-coloured bottle	8
	Red-coloured bottle	12		Red-coloured bottle	6
	Transparent bottle	8		Transparent bottle	4
	Sky blue, green-coloured bottle	4		Sky blue, green-coloured bottle	2
Red-coloured beer	Brown or dark-coloured bottle	12	Sky blue or green-coloured beer	Brown or dark-coloured bottle	4
	Red-coloured bottle	9		Red-coloured bottle	3
	Transparent bottle	6		Transparent bottle	2
	Sky blue, green-coloured bottle	3		Sky blue, green-coloured bottle	1

- The absorption of UV rays can be also demonstrated in coloured beverages: depending on the chosen colour or food additive, the amount of MBT will be increased
- Sky blue and green colours should allow a measurable absorption under 500 nm. Should these colours be added as food colourants in beers, the increase of MBT should be remarkably accelerated with or without the support of coloured or transparent bottles
- On the other hand, reddish colours should exhibit different behaviours. As reported in the literature, red wines appear less sensible to light because of higher tannin contents and the presumable production of pigmented tannins from anthocyanins and tannins [48].

As a consequence the best strategy should be the effective coupling of:

- A brown or dark-coloured beer (sky blue, green colours should be avoided), and
- A brown or dark-coloured glass bottle (transparent, sky blue, green tints should not be recommended).

On these bases, the comparison could be interpreted as shown in Table 4.1: the qualitative performance might be approximately calculated on the basis of this formula:

$$P = R_{beer} \times A_{glass}$$

where P = qualitative performance of IFP, R_{beer} = augmented risk of MBT production and A_{glass} means the approximate UV absorption of glass bottles.

P values are clearly indicative and have to be tested experimentally, but useful indications may be obtained. In addition, critical factors such as the dimension and the thickness of glass bottles have not been considered (Table 4.1). As a result, suggested results have to be necessarily validated because of the hypothetical meaning of obtained results: this approach is similar to the known 'Hazard Analysis and Critical Control Points' (HACCP) approach in the food industry.

With concern to preliminary calculations, is might be assumed that R_{beer} and A_{glass} can vary from 1 to 4 when speaking of dark or brown tints (score: 4), red colours (score: 3), transparent matters (score: 2), sky blue or green tints (score: 1).

In summary, the choice of transparent bottles may appear justified if brown, dark-coloured or red-coloured beers are used. On the other side, the bottling of sky blue- or green-coloured beers in transparent bottles should not be recommended. Coloured bottles may be always useful when speaking of coloured beers with the notable exception of sky blue and green-coloured beverages: the use of the same tint for bottles seems highly dangerous. As a result, sky blue and green colours should be avoided in both situations (maximum score: 4 points) because of the risk of notable UV absorption and enhanced MBT production. Similarly, the use of transparent bottles or light-coloured beers is questionable: calculable scores do not exceed 8.

4.4 Identification

Appellative functions and identification are strictly connected. The attention of consumers has to be initially addressed to the specific IFP and confirmed by means of the easy identification between the observed object and the researched good [49]. The process of identification may give unexpected results if the specific IFP is connected with a 'universal' but different brand [50].

Anyway, the main problem of identification is always correlated to the cultural heritage and behaviour of targeted consumers [22]. On the other side, the IFP may be linked to unknown brands: in these situations, IFP must 'speak' and communicate its own features to the consumer by means of known and widely accepted languages [9].

4.5 Persuasive Function

The identification of IFP cannot be the end of the decisional process. In fact, consumers may identify a peculiar food with the researched good; on the other hand, the good impression has to be confirmed by means of subliminal, detailed and persuasive messages [51]. Clearly, persuasion can be cooperatively obtained with different sensorial stimuli: colours, materials, shapes, dimension of printed letters, etc. [52].

Actually, the complex persuasive strategy is often linked to the peculiar food category [53]. On the other side, the different sensorial (and often irrational) stimuli are mainly mediated by FP and correlated with specific, subliminal and unequivocal meanings [9, 54]:

- The referential value is specifically linked to the relation between costs and benefits of consumer goods (another good name would be 'food quality'…)
- The easiness of usage
- The concept of food product (psychological and social implications)
- The hedonistic value.

Actually, FP can surely join both rational and irrational values with correlated sensorial stimuli: anyway, the aim is the persuasion of the final user.

4.6 Informative Function

The last function of modern FP is surely the transfer of useful information to final users.

First of all, printable information is imposed by legal requirements, depending on different countries and/or geographical locations. Information can appear placed in marginal areas. However, the correct and strategically effective graphic placement of related data on FP surfaces may become one of main features of the IFP [55, 56].

With relation to modern food and non-food packages, the management of information by means of tables, text blocks, icons and chromatic elements is one of crucial elements [27]. Moreover, FP are more and more integrated 'speaking books' for inexperienced users in the evolving social context of fast-foods an ready-to-eat products. In past times, so-called 'usage instructions' were perceived as accessory additions, but new consumers are not skilled in food cooking and other 'simple' culinary operations. As a result, correct and reliable usage instructions are needed [13]. Actually, this situation is also caused by the modi-fication of traditional foods: another face of the evolving society.

On these bases, it can be also assumed that (a) the lack of competence of final consumers and (b) technological and performance-related evolution of FP and IFP have really opened new communicative challenges: FP is the tangible speaking interface between food and consumer [5]. So, packages have to be self-explana-tory; in addition, they should:

- Minimise the cognitive effort of final users [29]
- Furnish important data without redundancy by means of new communication strategies; secondary information should be avoided [57]
- Offer reliable food safety information [19, 58]

- Avoid the redundancy of important data
- And finally become a real advertising medium [51]. The self-explanatory function is important especially with reference to particular targets and foods (example: baby formulations) when speaking of food hygiene.

An useful example of modern communication strategies may be shown by peculiar containers such as asymmetrical glass bottles for red wines (Sect. 3.5). With reference to these containers, the creation of particular symbols is generally focused on the communication by means of dedicated logos or printed labels. In the above-mentioned situation, the slanting and asymmetrical profile of glass bottles has been studied to facilitate handling and to optimise the horizontal stacking of packaging with increased stability when bottles are placed in a flat position. In addition, the central part of this FP has been designed for different labels according to communicative exigencies of awarded wine producers. As a consequence, the asymmetrical FP identifies the whole IFP among other wines in spite of the possible application of different labels.

With relation to bottled wines and similar beverages, the application of printed labels is normally accepted. This traditional practice may be useful because of the introduction of 'smart' packaging devices (Sect. 2.2.5.4). In fact, the main function of these systems is strictly correlated to the flow of visual information: consequently, IP devices may ameliorate usage performances of the whole IFP. Consequently, the product is allowed to show a minimal amount of information without sensorial redundancy, while resting useful data are communicated by other advertising media.

From the chemical and technological viewpoints, a few points may be discussed with concern to wine bottles. First of all, the digital processing and production of modern adhesive labels and information brochures is fundamental. Moreover, similar techniques have surely broadened current food marketing perspectives, including possible analytical methods. In fact, imaging analyses are the last evolution of digital editing software for graphic projects [25].

A useful application of imaging techniques may be linked to quality control operations in the industry of wines. In detail, the analytical comparison between different lots of the same product may be carried out by means of the digital evaluation of chromatic mutations after several months (Sect. 3.5).

Colours may be measured in different ways: spectroscopy is reliable enough [59]. The redox reaction of phenolic compounds with the phosphomolybdic-phosphotungstic acid (*Folin-Chiocalteu* reagent) may be used: as a result, a blue-coloured complex is produced in alkaline solutions. The quantitative amount of this complex is measured at 765 nm. In addition, anthocyanins also can be evaluated and expressed as malvidin-3-*O*-glucoside equivalents at 540 nm [59]. Another strategy is the colour and hue analysis by direct measurement of wine samples at wavelengths of 420, 520 and 620 nm. Alternatively, the colorimetric analysis of digital images is recommended by means of free software products for personal computers [29].

The colorimetric performance of wines may be examined with reference to the bottled content. However, possible variations may be detected because of incorrect storage and/or excessive light exposure (Sects. 3.5 and 4.3). The useful evaluation of quality control may be suggested with reference to the external part of IFP. Because of the chemical inertness of glass materials from the colorimetric viewpoint, the performance of photosensible components of the external FP should be related to adhesive labels. On these bases, it can be assumed that a simple colorimetric examination on adhesive and printed labels could be made [25] by means of:

- A high resolution-digital camera
- An exposure system with two 45°-inclined light sources
- One of the freely available imaging software systems for personal computers.

As a result, possible analytical differences between distinct bottles of the same lot (or different lots) could be simply anticipated and/or explained by means of the digital comparison between acquired images of photosensible labels. As shown in Sect. 4.3, the possible formation of sunlight off-flavour in light-exposed alcoholic beverages may be partially explained with the original abundance of the photosensitiser riboflavin [60]. On these bases, it may be assumed that the susceptibility of certain wines to light exposure may be predictable, on the basis of known riboflavin contents and established light exposure conditions.

By contrast, abnormal variations should be explained with additional factors including higher light exposure than expected, in terms of intensity or storage times. As a consequence, wine alterations should be linked to the contemporary discoloration of related labels because of the augment of light intensity [25]. Similar works are undoubtedly easier if the colorimetric mutation may be studied and evaluated in terms of wavelengths and areas.

It could be inferred that asymmetrical bottles for wines may show peculiar information about the chemical stability of bottled contents (Sect. 3.5.1) if adhesive labels are partially photosensible and their colorimetric appearance may be correlated to the discoloration of wines. This case study is presented in the next Section.

4.6.1 Food Product: Bottled Red Wine in Asymmetrical-Shaped Bottles with Photosensible Labels and Evaluation of UV Light

Red wines are subjected to important modifications of related chemical and physical profiles during their storage (Sect. 3.5.1).

When speaking of red wines instead of white products, the situation might appear more complex. Actually, the pigmentation of these products and the more general modification of physicochemical features depend on winemaking techniques: length of skin contact, temperature, presence of seeds, stems and enzymes, etc. These parameters can affect the extraction of phenolics into the fermenting juice before the final bottling with the consequent modification of the antioxidant activity of wines [61].

After vinification, all wines may change their chemical profiles (Sect. 3.5.1): this complex phenomenon, generally named 'wine ageing', is not entirely known at present depending on various factors [62]. One of the more interesting modifications appears related to the composition of anthocyanin-derived pigments and the variation of wine colours from the original purple-red to the final brick-red hue [63]. The total pigment content in red wines may be calculated from the total area of chromatograms concerning non-fractionated samples at 520 nm and expressed as malvidin-3-O-glucoside [63]. This compound decreases normally during time when wines are aged in barrels. Could this diminution be correlated with any type of 'intelligent' label? Should this correlation be workable, the adhesive label should be large enough and probably placed on the most part of the exposed glass surface.

4.6.2 Bottled Red Wines: Photosensible Labels

Unfortunately, reliable photosensible labels are not reported at present in the scientific literature for this type of product. From the designer's viewpoint, the use of similar systems is attractive; on the other side, these solutions appear difficultly workable.

In fact, three problems at least should be solved before proposing a workable and economically valuable solution:

(1) Photosensible labels should be realised on peculiar paper bases, with photosensitive inks or polymeric-based materials. At present, the realisation of photosensitive polymers with added carotenoids, chlorophylls or food-grade colourants [29, 64–67] could be also proposed. The importance of carotenoids is mainly correlated with the higher absorption between 420 and 520 nm

(2) Unfortunately, all above-mentioned solutions may not resist to the prolongated light exposure, while wine ageing is supposed to be 10–15 months at least

(3) In addition, the common opinion of final users is not always favourable when active or intelligent packaging systems are applied to packaged foods [29].

For these reasons, the realisation of peculiar bottles with photosensible labels may be designed and proposed, but the effective use of this FP is not recommended: after all, the decomposition of wine pigments is quite visible through transparent glass without the need of 'intelligent' labels. On the other side, the use of similar labels can be useful for research and study purposes. However, the discoloration of wines can be also examined by means of the simple immersion of filter papers into red wines for 20 s only and the digital acquisition of wetted papers after 5 min of drying at room temperature. Figure 4.3 shows the simulated diminution of the total pigment content in several red wines during bottle ageing versus time.

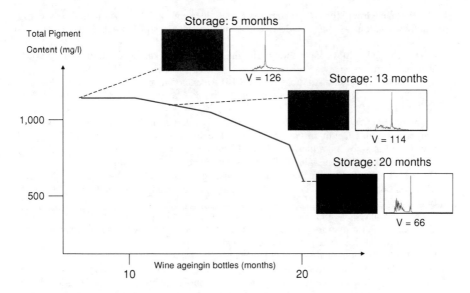

Fig. 4.3 The diminution of total pigments in bottled red wines during storage. This simulated *graph* shows the observable decrease. The diminution of the total pigment content (as malvidin-3-*O*-glucoside) can be measured with the colorimetric analysis of coloured filter papers after immersion in wine samples. The analysis can be performed by means of digital image and processing techniques on acquired pictures of paper specimens. For example, the *first picture* on the *upper side* concerns a peculiar red wine at 5 months of storage. The obtained pixel frequency histogram shows an average light intensity (V) of 126 at approximately 700 nm. After 20 months of storage, V is 66 at 700 nm: moreover, the correlated pixel frequency histogram shows also a certain dispersion of V values

Initial, intermediate and final tints are also displayed by means of three rect-angular images showing chromatic alterations on dried filter papers (images have been digitally acquired). The colorimetric measure of the light intensity (V)—of the red colour component (approximate wavelength of 700 nm) may be carried out with the analysis of acquired pictures [25]. With relation to a peculiar experiment, Fig. 4.3 shows that V values at 700 nm might decrease from 126 at 5 months of storage to 66 after 20 months. As a result, the colorimetric decrease can be easily shown without the use of photosensible labels. Figure 4.3 shows also three pixel frequency histograms for every acquired picture. A certain dispersion of V values (dark images) might be observed when V decreases.

References

1. Parisi S (2004) Alterazioni in imballaggi metallici termicamente processati. Gulotta Press, Palermo
2. Brunazzi G (2009) Hello! Logos. Logos, Modena

3. The Hartman Group, Inc (2013) Hartman Group: ideas in food 2013. A cultural perspective. http://www.hartman-group.com/downloads/white-papers/ideas-in-food-2013. Accessed 14 Dec 2013
4. Bozzola M (ed) (2011) Easy eating: sustainable paper packaging for traditional produce. Dativo, Milan
5. Vernuccio M, Cozzolino A, Michelini L (2010) An exploratory study of marketing, logistics, and ethics in packaging innovation. Eur J Innov Manag 13(3):333–354. doi:10.1108/14601061011060157
6. Shinkman M, Lewis P (2008) Rich pickings, opportunities in South-east Asia's emerging markets. Atradius Credit Insurance NV and The Economist Intelligence Unit, NY, p 15. http://www.asia-now.com/files/ideas/Rich%20pickings%20Opportunities%20in%20South%20East%20Asia's%20emerging%20markets.pdf. Accessed 28 Jan 2014
7. Guinee TP (2007) Introduction: what are analogue cheeses? In: McSweeney PLH (ed) Cheese problems solved. Woodhead Publishing Limited, Cambridge, and CRC Press LLC, Boca Raton, pp 384–386
8. Codex Alimentarius Commission (1995) Codex general standard for food additives, last revision 2013. Codex Alimentarius—International Food Standards. http://www.codexalimentarius.net/gsfaonline/docs/CXS_192e.pdf. Accessed 18 Oct 2013
9. Volli U (2012) Semiotica della pubblicità. Laterza, Rome
10. Fonseca SC, Oliveira FAR, Brecht JK, Chau KV (1999) Development of perforation-mediated modified atmosphere packaging for fresh-cut vegetables. In: Oliveira FAR, Oliveira JC (eds) Processing foods: quality optimization and process assessment. CRC Press, Boca Raton, p 392
11. Tanaka M (2009) Phthalocyanines—high performance pigments and their applications. In: Faulkner EB, Schwartz RJ (eds) High performance pigments, 2nd edn. Wiley–VCH, Weinheim, p 277
12. Piergiovanni L, Limbo S (2010) Materiali, tecnologie e qualità degli alimenti. Springer, Milan
13. Hartmann C, Dohle S, Siegrist M (2013) Importance of cooking skills for balanced food choices. Appetite 65(1):125–131. doi:10.1016/j.appet.2013.01.016
14. Petrini C (2009) Terra Madre. Come non farci mangiare dal cibo. Giunti, Florence
15. Food and Agriculture Organization of United Nations (2013) The state of food and agriculture 2013: food system for better nutrition. FAO. www.fao.org/docrep/018/i3300e/i3300e.pdf. Accessed 14 Dec 2013
16. Popkin BM, Adair LS, Ng SW (2012) Global nutrition transition and the pandemic of obesity in developing countries. Nutr Rev 70(1):3–21. doi:10.1111/j.1753-4887.2011.00456.x
17. Morris ER, Hill AD (1995) Inositol phosphate, calcium, magnesium, and zinc contents of selected breakfast cereals. J Food Compost Anal 8(1):3–11. doi:10.1006/jfca.1995.1002
18. Hartman Group (2013) Ideas in food. A cultural perspective. The Hartman Group, Inc. http://www.hartman-group.com/downloads/white-papers/ideas-in-food-2013. Accessed 14 Dec 2013
19. Disdier AC, Marette S (2013) Globalisation issues and consumers' purchase decisions for food products: Evidence from a laboratory experiment. Eur Rev Agric Econ 40(1):23–44. doi:10.1093/erae/jbr065
20. Bucchetti V (2005) Packaging design. Storia, linguaggi, progetto. Franco Angeli, Milan
21. Germak C (2008) Man at the centre of the project. Allemandi, Torino
22. De Nardo LM (2009) Food packaging: designing with the consumer. Elledì, Milan
23. Unander T, Nilsson H-E (2011) Evaluation of RFID based sensor platform for packaging surveillance applications. In: 2011 IEEE international conference on RFID-technologies and applications, RFID-TA 2011, Article no. 6068611, pp 27–31
24. Parisi S (2012) Food packaging and food alterations: the user-oriented approach. Smithers Rapra Technology, Shawbury
25. Parisi S (2013) Food industry and packaging materials—performance-oriented guidelines for users. Smithers Rapra Technology, Shawbury

26. Parisi S, Laganà P, Gioffrè ME, Minutoli E, Delia S (2013) Problematiche Emergenti di Sicurezza Alimentare. Prodotti Etnici ed Autenticità. In: Abstracts of the XXIV Congresso Interregionale Siculo Calabro SitI, Palermo, 21 23 June 2013. Euno Edizioni, Leonforte, ISBN: 978-88-97085-86-7

27. Ciravegna E (2010) La qualità del packaging. Franco Angeli, Milan

28. Bucchetti V (2007) Packaging contro-verso. Dativo, Milan

29. Olins W (1989) Corporate identity. Thames and Hudson, London

30. Bray C (ed) (2001) Dictionary of glass: materials and techniques, 2nd edn. University of Pennsylvania Press, Philadelphia, p 45

31. The European paper and board food packaging chain (2012) Industry guideline for the compliance of paper & board materials and articles for food contact, Issue 2 September 2012. In: Confederation of European paper industries (CEPI) and international confederation of paper (CITPA), Brussels

32. Robertson GL (ed) (2012) Food packaging: principles and practice, 3rd edn. CRC Press, Boca Raton, p 195

33. Pilley KP (1981) Lacquers, varnishes and coatings for food and drink cans and for the decorating industry. Arthur Holden Surface Coatings Ltd., Birmingham

34. Ottaviani F (2002) Il metodo HACCP (Hazard analysis and critical control points). In: Andreis G, Ottaviani F (eds) Manuale di sicurezza degli alimenti. Principi di ecologia microbica e di legislazione applicati alla produzione alimentare. Oxoid S.p.A., G. Milanese, Milan

35. De Keukeleire D (2000) Fundamentals of beer and hop chemistry. Quim Nova 23(1): 108–112. doi:10.1590/S0100-40422000000100019

36. Baglio E (2014) The modern yoghurt. Introduction to fermentative processes. In: Baglio E (ed) Chemistry and technology of yoghurt fermentation, SpringerBriefs in Chemistry of Foods. Springer International Publishing AG, Cham

37. Tucker GS (2003) Food biodeterioration and methods of preservation. In: Coles R, McDowell D, Kirwan MJ (eds) Food packaging technology. Blackwell Publishing Ltd, Oxford, pp 32–64

38. Brown H, Williams J (2003) Packaged product quality and shelf life. In: Coles R, McDowell D, Kirwan MJ (eds) Food packaging technology. Blackwell Publishing Ltd, Oxford

39. Page B, Edwards M, May N (2003) Metal cans. In: Coles R, McDowell D, Kirwan MJ (eds) Food packaging technology. Blackwell Publishing Ltd, Oxford

40. Girling PJ (2003) Packaging of food in glass containers. In: Coles R, McDowell D, Kirwan MJ (eds) Food packaging technology. Blackwell Publishing Ltd, Oxford

41. Kirwan MJ, Strawbridge JW (2003) Plastics in food packaging. In: Coles R, McDowell D, Kirwan MJ (eds) Food packaging technology. Blackwell Publishing Ltd, Oxford

42. Narziss L (1986) Technological factors of flavour stability. J Inst Brew 92(4):346–353. doi:10.1002/j.2050-0416.1986.tb04421.x

43. Vogler A, Kunkely H (1982) Photochemistry and beer. J Chem Educ 59(1):25–27. doi:10. 1021/ed059p25

44. Van Der Ark R, Blokker P, Bolshaw L, Brouwer ER, Hughes PS, Kessels H, Olierook F, Van Veen M (2011) Washington, DC: U.S. Patent and Trademark Office. Beverages and foodstuffs resistant to light induced flavour changes, processes for making the same, and compositions for imparting such resistance. US Patent 7,989,014, 2 Aug 2011

45. Palamand SR (1983) Method for controlling light stability in malt beverages and product thereof. US Patent 4,389,421, 21 Jun 1983

46. Irwin AJ, Barker RL, Pipast P (2001) Absorptive treatments for improved beer flavor stability. US Patent 6,207,208, 27 May 2001

47. Stewart GG (2004) The chemistry of beer instability. J Chem Educ 81(7):963–968. doi:10. 1021/ed081p963

48. Remy S, Fulcrand H, Labarbe B, Cheynier V, Moutounet M (2000) First confirmation in red wine of products resulting from direct anthocyanin–tannin reactions. J Sci Food Agric 80(6):745–751. doi:10.1002/(SICI)1097-0010(20000501)80:6<745:AID-JSFA611>3.0.CO;2-4

49. Ares G, Besio M, Gimenez A, Deliza R (2010) Relationship between involvement and functional milk desserts intention to purchase. Influence on attitude towards packaging characteristics. Appetite 55(2):298–304. doi:10.1016/j.appet.2010.06.016
50. Gelici-Zeko MM, Lutters D, Ten Klooster R, Weijzen PLG (2013) Studying the influence of packaging design on consumer perceptions (of dairy products) using categorizing and perceptual mapping. Packag Technol Sci 26(4):215–228. doi:10.1002/pts.1977
51. Margolin V (2013) Design studies and food studies: parallels and intersections. Des Cult 5(3):375–392. doi:10.2752/175470813X13705953612327
52. Riccò D (2008) Sentire il design. Sinestesie nel Progetto di Comunicazione. Carrocci, Rome
53. Bulmer S, Buchanan-Oliver M (2011) Brands as resources in intergenerational cultural transfer. Adv Cons Res 39:379–384. ISSN: 00989258
54. Pastore A, Vernuccio M (2004) Il packaging nel processo di consumo: prospettive di analisi tra Semiotica e Marketing. Finanz Mark Prod 3:108–137. ISSN: 1593-2230
55. MacRae R, Szabo M, Anderson K, Louden F, Trillo S (2012) Empowering the citizen-consumer: re-regulating consumer information to support the transition to sustainable and health promoting food systems in Canada. Sustainability 4(9):2146–2175. doi:10.3390/su4092146
56. Pereno A, Tamborrini P (2013) Packaging as a means for promoting sustainable and aware consumption. In: Proceedings of 4th international symposium on sustainable design, Federal University of Rio Grande do Sul, Porto Alegre, 12–14 November 2013
57. Boylston S (2009) Designing sustainable packaging. Laurence King Publishing Ltd., London
58. Eden S (2011) Food labels as boundary objects: how consumers make sense of organic and functional foods. Public Underst Sci 20(2):179–194. doi:10.1177/0963662509336714
59. Ivanova V, Dörnyei Á, Márk L, Vojnoski B, Stafilov T, Stefova M, Kilár F (2011) Polyphenolic content of Vranec wines produced by different vinification conditions. Food Chem 124(1):316–325. doi:10.1016/j.foodchem.2010.06.039
60. Mattivi F, Monetti A, Vrhovšek U, Tonon D, Andrés-Lacueva C (2000) High-performance liquid chromatographic determination of the riboflavin concentration in white wines for predicting their resistance to light. J Chromatogr A 888(1–2):121–127
61. Burns J, Gardner PT, Matthews D, Duthie GG, Lean J, Crozier A (2001) Extraction of phenolics and changes in antioxidant activity of red wines during vinification. J Agric Food Chem 49(12):5797–5808. doi:10.1021/jf010682p
62. Del Alamo Sanza M, Nevares Domínguez I (2006) Wine aging in bottle from artificial systems (staves and chips) and oak woods: anthocyanin composition. Anal Chim Acta 563(1):255–263. doi:10.1016/j.aca.2005.11.030
63. Alcalde-Eon C, Escribano-Bailón MT, Santos-Buelga C, Rivas-Gonzalo JC (2006) Changes in the detailed pigment composition of red wine during maturity and ageing: a comprehensive study. Anal Chim Acta 563(1):238–254. doi:10.1016/j.aca.2005.11.028
64. Bianchi RF, Schimitberger T, De Vasconcelos CKB, Ferreira GR (2010) Method for producing an intelligent label, intelligent label and uses thereof, method for preparing solutions in ampoules, solutions and compositions based on conjugated polymers, and electronic device for monitoring radiation doses. US Patent Application 13/512,717, 13 Dec 2012
65. Chappelle EW, Kim MS, McMurtrey JE III (1992) Ratio analysis of reflectance spectra (RARS): an algorithm for the remote estimation of the concentrations of chlorophyll a, chlorophyll b, and carotenoids in soybean leaves. Remote Sens Environ 39(3):239–247
66. Petersen M, Wiking L, Stapelfeldt H (1999) Light sensitivity of two colorants for Cheddar cheese. Quantum yields for photodegradation in an aqueous model system in relation to light stability of cheese in illuminated display. J Dairy Res 66(04):599–607
67. Zur Y, Gitelson AA, Chivkunova OB, Merzlyak MN (2000) The spectral contribution of carotenoids to light absorption and reflectance in green leaves. In: Proceedings of the 2nd international conference geospatial information in agriculture and forestry, Buena Vista, 10–12 January 2000, vol 2. http://digitalcommons.unl.edu/cgi/viewcontent.cgi?article=1274&context=natrespapers

Chapter 5
Packaging and Quality

Abstract Food packaging has to comply with complex requirements: functional implications, need of detailed information, regulatory obligations, impact on the environment. The disposal stage of packaging materials concerns many aspects, from the edible content (when it is not consumed) to the 'tertiary packaging' unit (it comprehends 'm' secondary packaging and 'n' packaged products). Best environmental strategies appear the numerical reduction of packaging components, the use of mono-material packages and the concomitant definition of 'ecodesign guidelines'. Consequently, recycling can be simplified and the possible reuse of recovered matters for food applications may be workable because of the limitation of chemical contamination. On the other side, economic worries and the full compliance with food safety requirements should be taken into account in the design step. The realisation of environmentally sustainable and food-contact approved packaging can be very challenging for all involved players.

Keywords Food packaging · Integrated food product · Remaining shelf life · Secondary packaging · Tertiary packaging · Ecodesign guidelines

Abbreviations

BPG	Best practice guideline
ETP	Electrolytic tin plate
FM	Food manufacturer
FP	Food packaging
FPP	Food packaging producer
GCC	Ground calcium carbonate
IFP	Integrated food product
MPU	Macro packaging unit
MAP	Modified atmosphere packaging
PCC	Precipitated calcium carbonate
RSL	Remaining shelf life
SPU	Secondary packaging unit
SDS	Sodium stearate

© The Author(s) 2014
G. Brunazzi et al., *The Importance of Packaging Design for the Chemistry of Food Products*, SpringerBriefs in Chemistry of Foods,
DOI: 10.1007/978-3-319-08452-7_5

5.1 Food Packaging and Environmental Ethics

Food packaging (FP) have to comply with complex requirements (Sect. 2.1); the design stage is specifically oriented to the satisfaction of heterogeneous needs: functional implications, necessity of detailed information, regulatory obligations, the specificity of packaged edible products.

In addition, food packaging wastes have a huge impact on the environment. In fact, most part of FP are "single-use' products with a short lifecycle: FP becomes waste at the end of shelf life of foods, with the exception of a few reusable pack [1].

Second, FP wastes concern following components of 'integrated food products' (IFP):

- The edible content (when it is not consumed)
- The primary packaging
- The secondary packaging (which contains 'n' IFP)
- The tertiary packaging (which contains 'm' secondary pack).

According to recent statistic data, every European citizen is supposed to produce about 156 kg of packaging wastes per year [2]. For these reasons, environmental requirements are extremely important for FP designers at present [3, 4].

With exclusive relation to edible products, the symbolic value and functional requirements of foods (Sect. 2.2) have a notable influence of FP and their environmental 'compatibility' [5, 6].

Differently from other product categories, two main features should be taken into account by FP designers: the perishability and the edibility of packaged foods [7, 8]. These prerequisites can be important for the satisfaction of functional and communicative requirements (Sects. 2.2 and 3.3); on the other side, national and international organisations require more and more significant efforts in favour of waste reduction. Of course, the best strategy would appear the numerical reduction of packaging production (according to weights, volumes and materials) but this approach should be shared between all interested 'stakeholders'.

For these reasons, the joint creation of common 'best practice guidelines' (BPG) would be warmly welcomed. The successive step should naturally be the implementation of BPG (with necessary adjustments) in every productive sector and subsector [9, 10].

Moreover, the creation and implementation of useful BPG has other important aims: first of all, the possibility of forecasting and preventing the future evolution of food microbial ecology and physicochemical profiles with correlated dangers for human health. Designers can operate with this approach if the expected use of FP is clearly defined. At present, more efforts appear still needed when speaking of correct cooperation between food manufacturers or packers (FM) on the one hand and food packaging manufacturers (FPP) on the other side [7].

5.1.1 Numerical Reduction of Packaging Units

Modern distributive systems are based on the transportation of notable amounts of food and non-food commodities by means of the logical and possibly ordered subdivision in macro-unities (Sect. 3.4). In other words, 'n' different FP with the same identification are included into a single secondary packaging unit (SPU) and 'm' of these SPU are subsequently assembled together with the aim of creating a single macro packaging unit (MPU). With the exception of MPU, it should be remembered that SPU have been progressively transformed in additional advertising materials (Sect. 3.4). However, environmentally sustainable strategies often require the reduction of final waste. As above mentioned, the simpler solution could be the numerical reduction of primary and secondary packages [5]. The reduction of FP implies that IPF should be redesigned because of the necessary increase of sizes and weights. As a result, mechanical performances and physicochemical modifications of packaged foods should be notably influenced with unknown results.

For this reason, it may be suggested that SPU are redesigned instead of FP despite the different attitude of primary and secondary packages with concern to reuse: FP are often disposable applications with one possible destiny only, while SPU may be easily reused in the commercial cycle.

Should the reduction of SPU be applied, new productive strategies would be considered with important consequences. First of all, the chemical composition of SPU constituents should be significantly modified. For example, the augment of SPU inner spaces can be considered but the natural consequence of this approach would be the parallel increase of thicknesses. As a clear result, normal advertising open SPU for food products (Sect. 3.4) could simply be larger than usual.

On the other hand, modified SPU should show increased mechanical performances: for example, compactness has to be assured and consequently enhanced. Indeed, larger paper boxes can contain more FP unities but mechanical tensions within the single SPU and between adjacent SPU have to be taken into account. For this reason, the use of adhesive products has to be considered because of the necessity of increased cohesive forces and chemical bonds between different paper layers (e.g. corrugated papers). Normally, several of most used adhesive products for paper and board packaging are [11]:

- Water-soluble glues. Generally, these products are starch or protein solutions. Additionally, rubber additives may be added. General uses: Uncoated and ink-coated paper supports
- Dispersion glues, also named 'white' glues. These products contain small polymeric particles. Resulting glues are correctly defined dispersions. Several additives may be present for helping wettability, paper softening and the final adhesion. Anyway, these glues are designed for medium or slow-speed operations and polyethylene- coated supports

- Hot-melt adhesives. Normally, the approximate composition involves thermoplastic polymers, other resins, waxes and antioxidant additives. These glues are usable for hot-melt processing (thermal ranges for applications are 100–200 °C). Basically, hot-melt adhesives are designed for high-speed operations.

Above-mentioned products have to be carefully chosen in the initial design step because of possible FP and IFP failures [7]. In fact, the formation of glue rivulets in the assembling of paperboard FP may be dangerous: normally, these failures are caused in processing steps (incorrect thermal values, too rapid operations, etc.), but rheological problems can also occur. Moreover, the possible migration of toxic substances (9,10-dihydroanthracene, retene, etc.) by hot-melt adhesives and other glues may be object of dedicated studies [12].

Another approach is related to the amount of mineral fillers. These substances, usually pigments, are added to the pulp for improving opacity [11]. However, this strategy should be carefully considered because of incorrect storage conditions: in fact, most used mineral fillers are recognised to have a hydrophobic nature; consequently, reduced additions of mineral fillers (or the use of unmodified fillers) may transform paperboard surfaces into hydrophilic materials with consequent paper damages and miniaturisation of packaged foods. Basically, mineral compounds may be found in the following list [13, 14]:

- Ground calcium carbonate (GCC),
- Precipitated calcium carbonate (PCC)
- Kaolin (also known as 'China clay') and calcinated kaolin
- Talc
- Titanium dioxide.

The presence of mineral fillers has to be highlighted in spite of the apparent lack of correlation with food safety. In fact, normal microbial contamination on paper and board packages may be highly favoured if FP are able to absorb notable quantities of water vapour. In addition, food chemical contamination may be also enhanced in these conditions [4, 7]. On the other hand, most used mineral fillers for paper and board FP–GCC, etc.—have a hydrophobic nature [14]. Actually, GCC is originally hydrophilic.

A dedicated surface modification is required in the preparation of GCC powders because the original calcium carbonate (hydrophilic particles) has to be compatible with plastics, rubber and adhesives. Consequently, hydrophilic GCC can be turned into hydrophobic particles after surface modification: for example, the addition of peculiar compounds like sodium stearate (SDS) and the concomitant wet ultra-fine grinding technique can be used with success [15].

Quality control of used fillers is crucial because of the necessity of using only hydrophobic pigments; moreover, quantitative additions of these mineral compounds have to be monitored constantly during the production.

5.1.2 Mono-material Packaging and Possible Separation into Basic Components

With relation to recycling activities, mono-material packages are normally preferred; another good choice is to collect only similar and compatible FP wastes in the recycling step. However, the easy transformation of multi-material FP in separated components is always advised and possibly communicated to the final user (normal food consumers).

Functional requirements have to be preliminarily taken into account in the design step (Sect. 2.2). On the other side, it should be noted that 'environmentally-friendly' prototypes have to comply with three different exigencies at the same time:

1. FP and the related IFP should be easily preserved, storable and transportable
2. Mechanical tensions, bumps, superficial damages, thermal variations should not alter packaged foods
3. Final packaging should be fit for every possible recovery procedure, including the preliminary disjunction of multi-material FP in separated components.

It has to be noted that above shown requirements may appear very challenging for designers: most part of FP are produced and delivered to FM or intermediate players in a well specified condition without similarity to the final aspect of IFP. For example, flexible films for dairy products are produced as single spools but the final product is naturally different (e.g. thermosealed FP for soft cheeses). In addition, FP can be assembled near FPP or FM with one or more components. As a result, FP should remain intact after use (in one specified shape or condition) and maintain same technical and chemical performances when the final IFP is assembled.

With the clear exception of mono-material packaging, the keypoint is the easy or difficult separation between:

- Plastic components and metallic supports (FP category: metal cans and similar products)
- Plastic and cellulosic parts (FP category: paper and board packaging)
- Plastic, metallic (where present) and cellulosic parts (FP category: composite systems)
- Glass (FP category: glass packaging) and cellulosic components with little amounts of plastic matters (accessory material: adhesive labels).

At present, glass packaging only appear easily recoverable but the total separation between heterogeneous components of the same FP should be demonstrated. In fact, glass FP is normally destined to be melted. The percentage of extraneous compounds may appear negligible and related to the presence of adhesive residues by printed labels [16]. For this reason, extraneous substances do not seem to influence the quality of recovered materials and the technological performance of final FP by virgin and recycled glass [1]. Probably, the most important fraction of extraneous matters originates from metallic or plastic caps; however, these components are generally absent in the recycling step.

With the exception of glass packaging, remaining FP do not seem to be easily separable in single components. Moreover, it should be highlighted that:

- Every single mono-material and homogenous FP component is normally subdivided in different sub-parts
- The concomitant presence of dissimilar materials in the macroscopic composition of assembled FP can be questionable from the hygienic viewpoint.

For example, a common three-piece metal can (basic support: electrolytic tin plate) correspond to the stratification of following materials (the below displayed list is not exhaustive):

- Metallic components:

  - Electrolytic tin plate (ETP); steel or aluminium parts (for 'easy-open end' rings)
  - Copper oxide on longitudinal sealing areas

- Plastic components:

  - Epoxyphenolic coatings or enamels (food-contact inner side): this product contains also inorganic pigments like titanium dioxide
  - Lithographic system on the external side (the stratification of 'n' different printing inks, where $n = 1$ or more inks); every ink contains inorganic or organic pigments
  - Primary external coating (under the lithographic system, printed or 'neutral' external side)
  - Finishing (also named 'transparent' or 'over') coating: it protects the whole lithographic system on the external side
  - Inner gasket (it is located into inner edges of can tops and covers)
  - Side seam coating (on the longitudinal sealing area).

Similar products cannot be separated. As a consequence, metal cans may be recovered and recycled by fusion, for example. Clearly, recycled materials can contain negligible amounts of organic and heterogeneous nature. However, the utilisation of similar 'raw materials' for FP productions may be questionable because of food contamination episodes (e.g. mineral oils, organic residues by ink combustion, etc.) [4]. On the other hand, the same recovered and recycled material could be used to produce packaging for non-food applications.

5.1.3 Packaging Life Cycle Extension

With relation to the reduction of FP wastes, designers can also propose reusable packaging and single components with extended life cycles. Naturally, this approach is environmentally-oriented: designers and FPP should also combine the attention to 'good recycling practices' with food safety and consumers' interests. In other words, the design activity has to take into account all requirements including the possible occurrence of public health dangers: theoretically, the hypothetical number of food hygiene failures should be directly proportional to the number of consecutive FP reuses. The same thing can be supposed when speaking of mechanical performances and chemical inertness. For example, normal food-contact approved plastic boxes for household application might show too oiled surfaces or superficial damages after a certain number of washing treatments.

Similar compositions show also the presence of plasticisers: the simple ethylene glycol is one of known examples [7]. Consequently, lubricates surfaces may be explained because of:

- Superficial damage of plastic packaging, and/or
- Partial transfer of food lipids on plastic surfaces and permanent adsorption (fatty molecules are often good lubricants).

In addition, plastic materials are normally subjected to the natural 'ageing': this term means that many polymers are progressively modified with reference to physicochemical composition. For example, the oxidation of certain polymers is a form of chemical ageing. Because of the possibility of accelerated reactions, ageing speed may be remarkable in several situations: probably, the continuous reuse of household food packaging is one of the most important causes of accelerated ageing with relation to the effect of different chemical attacks to polymeric structures and dispersed additives such as plasticisers [7].

5.1.4 Reduction of Weights and Sizes

Sometimes, communicative strategies aim to enforce the apparent perception of food quantities by means of oversized packaging, similarly to other non-food products. For example, most part of software products are presented and sold into really oversized boxes if compared with the real dimension of technological supports.

On the other side, fresh foods are often packaged into large packaging because of the limited availability of FP sizes. As above stated, designers may also reduce dimensional properties of FP: this strategy is completely different from the approach of Sect. 5.1.1.

Dimensionally-reduced FP should have different compositions: for this reason, the reduction of weights and volumetric capacities should be carefully studied because of edible contents.

Usually, reduced FP sizes imply also reduced thicknesses: so the resulting IFP may show some sensorial modification [17]. In fact, the reduced thickness may explain micro-fractures or similar FP damages in 'modified atmosphere packaging' (MAP) vegetables because of the continuous modification of the inner gaseous composition [18].

With reference to microbial spreading, MAP systems have been introduced for fresh-cut fruit and vegetable products with the aim of extending 'remaining shelf life' (RSL) values. This objective can be obtained by reducing water losses, microbial spreading, ethylene biosynthesis and other factors, including also so-called 'respiration' rates [19].

With concern to respiration, this term is referred to the visible result of oxidative reactions in living organisms, including also vegetables: in detail, lipids and carbohydrates are oxidised to carbon dioxide and water [20]. Respiration is still active in fresh cut and minimally processed vegetables: at present, the most successful strategy for the reduction of respiration rates and the resulting RSL enhancement is offered by MAP technology. However, respiration rates can be different depending on packaged vegetables and inner gaseous mixtures; moreover, used films and plastic boxes or trays may show different permeability values. These factors surely influence the design of FP [19]: in fact, low oxygen quantities in the inner atmosphere may promote anaerobic fermentation in ready-to-eat products with dangerous consequences. Packages should assure acceptable volumetric sizes because of the necessity of storing enough oxygen into MAP products. Should this preliminary condition not be satisfied, different vegetables (mushrooms, broccoli, etc.) with notable respiration rates would cause the rapid consumption of the available oxygen with resulting anaerobic fermentation before expiration dates. Clearly, anaerobiosis may imply toxin formation by anaerobic pathogens. In addition, high respiration rates may cause the rapid collapse of MAP boxes or trays if used films and rigid packaging are sufficiently permeable to carbon dioxide and water vapour [18].

Naturally, collapsed FP lose the original integrity with other problems [21]:

- Seal rupture, fractures on trays and boxes, etc.
- Environmental contamination (external toxicants may permeate damaged films, boxes and trays)
- Insect contamination
- Foreign bodies (wooden fragments, etc.)
- Microbial contamination
- And the natural modification of the inner atmosphere.

5.1.5 Environmentally Sustainable Labelling

IFP may show and communicate information of interest in two ways:

- The use of previously printed FP is often considered. Alternatively,
- 'Neutral' packaging or the association of non-printed packaging components may be used and subsequently provided with printed adhesive labels.

The first solution appears the most logical choice; however, marketing strategies and commercial agreements may advice different approaches. For example, a peculiar IFP may be produced with a determined brand by a specified FP.

However, FP can produce the same type of food product with other brands by permission, including its own name.

Usually, 'n' different brands should require 'n' printed FP or printed components: this situation may be economically unacceptable if the production of one or more of 'n' different IFP has to be stopped after a specified number of months. This is the situation of current 'food auctions': a private label manager can announce one or more auctions with the aim of selecting best available FP on the market.

On the other hand, these 'commercial competitions' can force FP to produce the peculiar product until a determined temporal limit. As a consequence, FP have to preliminarily forecast and monitor the use of remaining FP or related components before the specified limit. In this situation, the storage of 'n' branded materials may be economically unacceptable because remaining FP could be used for the specified brand only.

So 'n' branded IFP may be packaged with non-printed and white o transparent (also named 'neutral') FP. Should this approach be considered, the subsequent step would be the use of printed adhesive labels on 'neutral' IFP. From the economic viewpoint, this choice is surely acceptable. On the other hand, similar strategies are not useful when speaking of environmentally sustainable packaging and easy separation of different FP components before recycling [22].

5.2 Packaging, Quality and Total Sustainability

Environmentally sustainable FP can easily communicate their enhanced quality to consumers. On the other hand, environmental requirements should be inserted in the initial design plan with other factors. It can be assumed that above mentioned strategies—reduction of sizes, use of recyclable materials with low 'ecological rucksack' values, etc.—are useful guidelines for FPP and FP when speaking of environmental sustainability [23]. However, 'sustainable' FP design should take into several factors [24]:

- Food-related performances (the IFP is the 'active subject)
- Food packaging-related performances
- Recycling requirements
- Marketing requirements
- Logistic needs
- Interactions between different stakeholders along the whole food chain
- Interactions between IFP, FP and the destination of wastes in terms of geographical location (e.g. possibility of reliable recovery, recycling; reusability of secondary packages, etc.).

In other words, sustainable design does not 'build' the idea of FP only on environmental or food-related bases: should this be the situation, final packaging could only be perceived as experimental prototypes or case studies. By contrast, all requirements have to be considered: functionality, communication, regulatory, environmental sustainability and real disposal possibilities with relation to the final geographical location [25]. Clearly, the rediscovery of ethnic and regional food excellences can also be adequately promoted by means of environmentally sustainable and local FP and IFP [26].

References

1. Italian Institute of Packaging (2013) Linee guida per la valutazione dell'idoneità al contatto con alimenti del packaging realizzato con materiale proveniente da riciclo. The Italian Institute of Packaging, Milan
2. Eurostat (2013) Packaging waste statistics. http://epp.eurostat.ec.europa.eu/statistics_explained/index.php/Packaging_waste_statistics. Accessed 17 Dec 2013
3. Barbero S, Cozzo B (2009) Ecodesign. H. F Ullmann, Königswinter
4. Vollmer A, Biedermann M, Grundböck F, Ingenhoff J-E, Biedermann-Brem S, Altkofer W, Grob K (2011) Migration of mineral oil from printed paperboard into dry foods: survey of the German market. Eur Food Res Technol 232:175–182. doi:10.1007/s00217-010-1376-6
5. Tamborrini P (2009) Design sostenibile. Oggetti, sistemi e comportamenti. Electa, Milan
6. Hanss D, Böhm G (2012) Sustainability seen from the perspective of consumers. Int J Consum Stud 36(6):678–687. doi:10.1111/j.1470-6431.2011.01045.x
7. Parisi S (2012) Food packaging and food alterations: the user-oriented approach. Smithers Rapra Technology, Shawbury
8. Marsh K, Bugusu B (2007) Food packaging—roles, materials, and environmental issues. J Food Sci 72(3):39–55. doi:10.1111/j.1750-3841.2007.00301.x
9. Manzini E, Vezzoli C (1998) Lo sviluppo di prodotti sostenibili. I requisiti ambientali dei prodotti industriali. Maggioli, Rimini
10. Tamborrini P, Barbero S (eds) (2013) Il Fare Ecologico. Il prodotto industriale e i suoi requisiti ambientali. Edizione Ambiente, Milan
11. Iggesund Paperboard AB (2006) Iggesund Paperboard Reference Manual. 4. Printing and converting performance. http://www.iggesund.com/Global/Iggesund%20documents/Paperboard%20documents/Iggesund%20Anchor%20Material/Reference%20manual/Reference%20manual%20Printing%20and%20converting%20performance.PDF. Accessed 03 Feb 2014
12. Vera P, Aznar M, Mercea P, Nerín C (2011) Study of hotmelt adhesives used in food packaging multilayer laminates. Evaluation of the main factors affecting migration to food. J Mater Chem 21:420–431. doi:10.1039/c0jm02183k
13. Gill RA Sr, Haskins WJ, Ingram EL (2002) New developments in PCC offer board improvements with economy. Pap Board Ind 2(4):30–31. http://www.specialtyminerals.com/fileadmin/user_upload/smi/Publications/S-PA-AT-PB-57.pdf. Accessed 03 Feb 2014
14. Grönfors J (2010) Use of fillers in paper and paperboard grades. Thesis Dissertation, Tampere University of Applied Sciences. http://www.theseus.fi/bitstream/handle/10024/16226/Gronfors_Jarkko.pdf?sequence=1. Accessed 03 Feb 2014
15. Ding H, Lu SC, Deng YX, Du GX (2007) Mechano-activated surface modification of calcium carbonate in wet stirred mill and its properties. Trans Nonferrous Met Soc China 17(5):1100–1104. doi:10.1016/s1003-6326(07)60232-5
16. Onusseit H (2006) The influence of adhesives on recycling. Res. Cons. Recyc. 46(2):168–181. doi:10.1016/j.resconrec.2005.05.009
17. Parisi S (2004) Alterazioni in imballaggi metallici termicamente processati. Gulotta Press, Palermo

18. Micali M, Parisi S, Minutoli E, Delia S, Laganà P (2009) Alimenti confezionati e atmosfera modificata. Caratteristiche basilari, nuove procedure, applicazioni pratiche. Ind Aliment 489·35–43

19. Gorny JR (1997) A summary of CA and MAP requirements and recommendations for fresh-cut (minimally processed) fruits and vegetables. In: Gorny JR (ed) Proceedings of seventh international controlled atmosphere conference, vol 5., Postharvest Outreach ProgramUniversity of California, Davis, pp 30–66

20. Mattos LM, Moretti CL, Ferriera MD (2012) Modified atmosphere packaging for perishable plant products. In: Dogan F (ed) Polypropylene, ISBN: 978-953-51-0636-4, InTech. http://www. intechopen.com/books/polypropylene/modified-atmosphere-for-perishable-plant-products. Accessed 30 Feb 2014

21. Hotchkiss JH (1995) Safety considerations in active packaging. In: Rooney ML (ed) Active food packaging. Springer, Dordrecht, p 239. doi: 10.1007/978-1-4615-2175-4_11

22. Ciravegna E (2010) La qualità del packaging. Franco Angeli, Milan

23. Boylston S (2009) Designing sustainable packaging. Laurence King Publishing Ltd., London

24. Bistagnino L (ed) (2011) Systemic design: designing the productive and environmental sustainability. Slow Food Editore, Bra. ISBN: 9788884992796

25. Germak C (2008) Man at the centre of the project. Allemandi, Torino

26. Bublitz MG, Peracchio LA, Andreasen AR, Kees J, Kidwell B, Miller EG, Motley CM, Peter PC, Rajagopal P, Scott ML, Vallen B (2013) Promoting positive change: advancing the food well-being paradigm. J Bus Res 66(8):1211–1218. doi:10.1016/j.jbusres.2012.08.014